THE SACRED TRADITION OF YOGA

श्री:

DR. SHANKARANARAYANA JOIS

The Sacred Tradition of YOGA

TRADITIONAL PHILOSOPHY,
ETHICS,
and
PRACTICES
for a
MODERN SPIRITUAL
LIFE

SHAMBHALA
BOSTON & LONDON
2015

SHAMBHALA PUBLICATIONS, INC.
Horticultural Hall
300 Massachusetts Avenue
Boston, Massachusetts 02115
www.shambhala.com

9 8 7 6 5 4 3 2 1

FIRST SHAMBHALA EDITION

Printed in the United States of America

♾ This edition is printed on acid-free paper that meets the American National Standards Institute z39.48 Standard.

♻ This book is printed on 30% postconsumer recycled paper.
For more information please visit www.shambhala.com.
Distributed in the United States by Penguin Random House LLC and in Canada by Random House of Canada Ltd

Designed by Michael Russem

LIBRARY OF CONGRESS CATALOGING-IN-PUBLICATION DATA
Jois, Shankaranarayana, author.
The sacred tradition of yoga: philosophy, ethics, and practices for a modern spiritual life / Dr. Shankaranarayana Jois.
pages cm
ISBN 978-1-61180-172-9 (paperback)
1. Yoga. I. Title
B132.Y6J624 2015
181'.45—dc23
2014017616

In memory of Sri Lakshminarayana Jois and Smt. Honnamma

This book is dedicated to the Divine Mother,
Śrī Śrī Vijayalakṣmī Śrī Mātā,
of Aṣṭāṅga Yoga Vijñāna Mandiram
Whose blessings have enabled me to proceed on the Yogic path.

Contents

Foreword

TODAY, yoga is increasingly being accepted all over the world. Because of its comprehensive nature and the many practical benefits it has to offer, vast numbers of people are beginning to practice various yogic disciplines. Even in India, where yoga first originated, there is renewed interest. However, for many Indians, yoga is still part of daily life.

Yogic techniques have undergone an evolution since ancient times. Many people have tried to adapt these teachings to the modern lifestyle. As a result, new techniques and styles of yoga have emerged everywhere. Teachers today are using their own interpretation of yogic concepts to develop their own teaching methodologies. This has certainly resulted in some good. Many people have benefited by living a healthier physical life. At the same time, many of the original teachings and techniques have been lost. Practices like āsana, prāṇāyāma, and other essential teachings have lost their original significance and purpose. Moreover, these deviations propagate the wrong impression about the real purpose of yoga.

In this context, Dr. K. L. Shankaranarayana Jois, an experienced and knowledgeable expert in yoga, has made a bold attempt to give the serious student of yoga a clear explanation of the fundamental concepts of yoga in this valuable work. Dr. Jois's work does not represent yoga from a particular school or philosophy. Rather, Jois introduces both basic and advanced elements of yoga, interweaving in-depth descriptions of practices, states of mind, ancient legends, anticipated questions, and meaningful experiences of the author himself.

According to the ancient seers and yogis, bliss is the ultimate goal of life. This is yoga. Dr. Jois teaches that our life is meant to experience this eternal bliss. He explains that this is the original nature of humankind, which has been completely forgotten. Becoming reacquainted with our true nature requires effort and practice. Specific techniques that will help us most depend on our individual constitution. To fully understand the complexity of all this requires an in-depth explanation of yoga. This unique work offers that explanation, ultimately focusing on the path of Aṣṭāṅga Yoga. The first two limbs—the ancient organizational format for these teachings—of the eight-limbed Aṣṭāṅga path are dealt with here in great detail. The magnanimity of these concepts is presented effectively in the context of developing an ideal yogic lifestyle. For genuine aspirants of yoga, a close study of *The Sacred Tradition of Yoga* will provide a strong foundation.

I hope Dr. Jois will follow this book with equally thorough and insightful writings on the remaining six limbs of Aṣṭāṅga Yoga.

Dr. Ganapathi Jois, HMSc,
PGDip in Yoga Therapy, PhD
Kasturba Medical College, Karnataka, India

Introduction from a Western Student

IT IS WITH great honor that I write an introduction to a book such as this. To read this book is to be in the company of someone who knows whereof he speaks, someone who has devoted his life, without reservation, to the quest for understanding and toward the goal of Realization. Although I can only comment from a Western perspective, I believe this book will be a valuable resource for those practitioners—both from the West and the East—who have set out on a yogic journey.

Over nearly twenty years, I have had the privilege to be among a small, but now growing, number of students who study periodically with Dr. Jois. Since my very first meeting with him, in 1997, I have been greatly awed by the depth of his knowledge and experience. Dr. Jois is a unique teacher and writer in today's marketplace of yoga. He is a humble man who takes on his responsibility as a teacher with the utmost seriousness and dedication. He does not seek new students but sees it as his duty to offer what he knows to those who wish to learn. *The Sacred Tradition of Yoga* now offers the world an opportunity to experience the treasured knowledge and insights he has to share.

Navigating a yogic path in today's modern world can be a challenging undertaking, regardless of whether you live in the West or the East. The world we live in is filled with materialistic distractions that disturb both our mind and body. Dr. Jois presents us with a vision of the ultimate goal of yoga and directs us toward the available tools we can use to reach that goal. Rather than a set of esoteric practices and disciplines, Dr. Jois presents clear and practical guidance to help us both understand and hopefully experience for ourselves why such practices and disciplines are truly meaningful.

Dr. Jois's central message throughout the book repeatedly underscores the great benefits we can gain from adopting a yogic lifestyle. This book can help us gradually integrate yogic practices and disciplines into our daily modern lives so as to become firmly established in such a lifestyle. Its promise is nothing less than access to the real and indescribable joy that yogic experience can offer us.

Some of these teachings may give rise to skepticism in the Western student who has been thoroughly trained to think critically, and who may be particularly sensitive in our current age of fundamentalist tendencies. To such students I would say that Dr. Jois brings new understanding to the importance of honoring the ancient traditions. Rather than suggesting that we blindly follow some prescription from the past, Dr. Jois challenges us to experience for ourselves the truth and joy that results from following these practices. Moreover, he challenges us to use our analytical mind to assess their usefulness and benefit in our daily lives.

That said, Dr. Jois's teachings offer specific explanations and directives that promise sublime fruits—as long as such practices are followed with a degree of seriousness and commitment. He encourages us all—Westerners and Indians alike—that we may experience the goal of Realization and Liberation, provided our approach is genuine and our effort is earnest.

I feel it is extremely rare today to encounter such a clear voice offering such authentic yogic teachings. Dr. Jois's mastery of the Saṃskṛta language is one of many keys he holds to unlock innumerable doors to the ancient Indian arts and sciences. To read his words and grasp his keen and nuanced understanding of the ancient texts is to experience a direct link to the enormous wisdom ancient India has to offer. This book is an immensely valuable compendium of this ancient and sacred tradition—designed for those who have a strong sense of connection and commitment to the yogic path.

I thank Dr. Jois for writing this book and sharing his experience and knowledge.

P. Conrad Zehrer
Sebastopol, California

Preface

TODAY WE SEE a great scarcity of human qualities such as contentment, happiness, peace, generosity, and the like. At the same time, qualities like egotism, ignorance, greed, jealousy, and hatred have all carved a place in the human heart. This imbalance has resulted in an abundance of misery and unhappiness throughout the world. It is the responsibility of all beings, especially those who feel these effects deeply within their hearts, to struggle hard to restore balance in our world. This work must begin with each individual, as the source of this misery lies within the individual alone.

Yoga is both a science and an art. It purifies the human system and fosters many noble qualities. It has been imparted by great sages for millennia and offers a comprehensive way to rediscover an ideal way of life. In this sense, the increasing popularity of yoga is very hopeful. There is a tremendous amount of information to be discussed about yoga, and it could not possibly be presented in one book. This book aims to highlight only some of the key philosophical and practical elements. This initial volume will offer a general introduction to yoga, as well as a detailed discussion of the first two limbs of Aṣṭāṅga Yoga—the yamas and niyamas. The remaining six limbs of Aṣṭāṅga Yoga: āsana, prāṇāyāma, pratyāhāra, dhāraṇā, dhyāna, and Samādhi, will be dealt with in subsequent volumes.

Perhaps the most important thing to bear in mind while reading this book is that the wisdom of yoga presented here originally evolved thousands of years ago in a very different society. We can surmise from the ancient literature and teachings that the ideals advocated by yoga were comparatively easier to implement in those days. We believe this was because of the receptive nature and encouragement of society and, most important, the great purity of mind found in seekers at that time. It is important to remember that we are now living in the Kali Yuga, an age in which humankind is highly extroverted and conditions are very challenging for yogic enlightenment.

One should keep in mind throughout the study of this material that what is presented in this book is a model for an *ideal* way of life in an *ideal* society. Let me encourage the reader to avoid feeling that he or she must adopt every idea presented here. Nor should anyone feel that he or she must embrace any of these ideals fully. Rather, a measured approach is the best way to begin.

Yoga as a whole provides a blueprint for a practitioner to attain union with the Eternal Truth, thereby attaining Realization and Liberation. For the purposes of this text, the word *Realization* means identifying with the true, or higher, Self. This is an experience of the Eternal Truth, God, or Brahma while in a transcendental state. *Liberation* refers to the freedom we gain from the misery caused by the birth-death-birth cycle once we merge with the Eternal Truth.

The text also suggests that the seeker find a Realized teacher to help him or her reach yogic states. This too is suggested as an ideal approach. Obviously, finding a Realized teacher may not be possible for a number of reasons, including the difficulty of determining who is truly Realized. However, the great yogi and sage Patañjali explained that Īśvara (the Supreme) Himself is the ultimate teacher for all. Through Nature, the seeker will also receive guidance from the Great Light and should not be discouraged if a Realized teacher cannot be found.

Yoga is available to people everywhere in this world; it is not limited to any creed, class, or gender. While written with a Western audience in mind, this book is intended for both Indian and non-Indian students—particularly enthusiastic and sincere seekers. At times, examples presented in the text may be more appropriate for a Western reader to grasp an idea; other times, the examples and stories may speak more clearly to an Indian reader. Some information will inevitably appear culturally specific to Indians, simply because yoga is historically and culturally rooted in India. The great yogis of the past viewed all sixty-four wings of Indian arts and sciences as originating from this human mind and body. Properly understood, these wings of knowledge are considered paths for Realization. Given that Indian culture itself is a product of these arts and sciences, it is thus the offspring of yoga applied to life. Therefore, while explaining practical aspects of yoga, we inevitably use examples from Indian culture.

This book may be particularly useful to individuals beginning a yoga practice and those who may not have an in-depth understanding of yoga. The subject of yoga is vast, and one may go into great detail in any given area. However, in an effort not to overwhelm a new practitioner, we have tried to strike a balance in the amount of detail presented on various concepts and explanations. I ask forgiveness if I fail to accurately or fully communicate the intended teachings.

We have taken several measures to make the text more accessible to the average reader. For this reason, we have mixed our references to the two genders throughout the book. The reader is free to use the gender-specific pronoun he or she chooses.

To help with proper pronunciation of all Saṃskṛta words and phrases, we have transliterated from Saṃskṛta following standard diacritical usage. We have also transliterated the names of historical and literary figures, as well as deities. For example, this means that the sage Vyasa is spelled Vyāsa and the God Rama is spelled Rāma. We hope this will remind or instruct readers to pronounce these particular names where the long "a" vowel is pronounced "aaah," whereas the short "a" is pronounced "ah" as in "father." A simple Samskrta pronunciation guide appears in the appendix.

Exceptions to this are the proper names of known places and twentieth-century people, which we left without diacritic markings to avoid confusion. Thus, we write of Hrishikesh rather than Hṛṣikeś and Ramana Maharshi rather than Ramaṇa Maharṣi. We apologize if this causes any difficulty or confusion and hope it simply increases an appreciation for this greatly honored and divine language.

All Saṃskṛta terms will be italicized when they are first introduced in the text; from thereon, they will not be italicized. We have also included an index at the end of the book for readers to crosscheck where words are defined and used throughout the text.

If a reader feels that certain concepts have been clarified and he or she has gained a greater understanding of the scope of and possibilities inherent in yoga, if he or she feels inspired to try and preserve this great tradition, or is drawn to learn more about the ideal yogic way of life, then this book will have succeeded in its intention. Furthermore, if the reader's heart is drawn to choose one or two of the ideas presented here and begin to gently implement them into his or her own lifestyle, then the expectations of this author have been exceeded.

With humble and sincere gratitude,

Dr. Shankaranarayana Jois

Acknowledgments

IN HOLY MEMORY of the lotus feet of the Eternal Teacher, I wish to express my gratitude to a few important people and events in my life that have led me to this particular juncture. I feel very thankful to those who, through their conscious or unconscious actions, have sown the seeds of an ideal lifestyle within me. Their kindheartedness is the true inspiration for writing this book.

The very first influence was my beloved father, Lakshminarayana Jois, who raised me in accordance with the ideal yogic way of life. He introduced me to Saṃskṛta study at a very early age and encouraged me to pursue a broad education that included the study of yoga.

Next, during my secondary education, I was initiated into the yogic limbs of āsana, prāṇāyāma, and ṣaṭkarma by a revered teacher, Narasinga Rao, who impressed me with his disciplined life and with his teachings. Though I was not able to capture all his teachings, he ignited a spark of interest in me that has continued to evolve in my life. For this, I am most thankful.

Later, during my Saṃskṛta studies at the Maharaja's Government Saṃskṛta College of Mysore, I had the opportunity to practice āsana and prāṇāyāma with Vidwan K. Pattabhi Jois, head of the Department of Yogic Sciences at the college. He taught me āsana and prāṇāyāma for nearly six years, and I cannot forget the love and affection he showed me.

Subsequently, I studied many of the original yogic texts and was motivated to learn the core of yoga during my college studies. At this time, I was introduced to the teachings of Śrī Raṅga Mahāguru, passed to me through his disciples. It was through this meaningful connection that I was able to study, understand, and appreciate yoga in a very in-depth and comprehensive way. This book is an expression of my sincere gratitude to the elderly disciples of Śrī Raṅga Mahāguru, including Vidwans Śrī Sheshachala Sharma, Śrī Ramabhadracharya, Śrī S. V. Chamu, Śrī Chayapati, Śrī Doreswamy, Śrī Ganesha Rao, Śrī Vijayanandakanda, Śrī Ramakrishna Gurudas, and others. In addition,

I want to express my gratitude to Paramahamsa Parivrajakacharya Śrī Śrī Ranga Priya Swamiji.

Most important, I wish to express my deepest gratitude to the great yogi Śrī Raṅga Mahāguru (1913–1969), a most honorable personage of this age. This Eternal Teacher, through his experience with the Divine, gained yogic sight, singular intelligence, and reflective tendencies, discovered the hidden layers of Truth in the human body and in the cosmos. This great yogi fully comprehended the real meaning of yoga practice and imparted it to the world with love and affection.

It is needless to say that many have supported and encouraged the undertaking of bringing this book (both first and second editions) to the public. I wish to express my heartfelt gratitude to the late Mr. N. Srikanta, who reviewed the first edition and suggested many important corrections and improvements. I extend my deepest gratitude, with salutations, to my Eternal Teacher Śrī Śrī Vijayalakṣmī Śrī Mātā, who released the first edition of this book, by her lotus hands, with blessings and affection, on the sacred day of Mahā Śivarātri in 2004.

I am very thankful for everyone who has extended their kind cooperation in bringing forth a revised second edition that comes closer to meeting our standards. In particular, I wish to thank Noelle Oxenhandler for her insightful critique and skillful editing. I also wish to thank Dr. Ganapathi Jois, who dedicated his time to reading the manuscript and providing a very helpful foreword for our readers.

Last, I offer a very special thanks to my wife, G. Vijaya, for the patience, cooperation, and support she rendered in the writing of this text from beginning to end.

Dr. Shankaranarayana Jois

PART ONE

YOGABHŪMIKĀ

The Foundation of Yoga

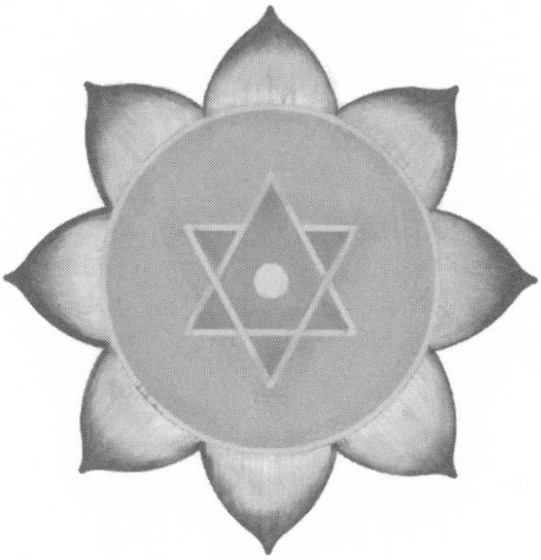

bhūmikā: earth, foundation; a small piece of earth; ***yogabhūmikā:*** the small piece of earth that has brought about yoga, known as *Bhārata,* or India

CHAPTER ONE

THE PURPOSE OF HUMAN LIFE

पुरुषार्थः

I WAS BORN in a small village in the south Indian state of Karnataka by the name of Konandoor. At that time, this village had no electricity and no motor vehicles. At the early age of three, I was taken from this village to the home of my maternal grandmother in Shimoga. My grandmother was a very spiritual person and spent many hours each day chanting prayers. She was a devoted woman with firm principles, and often her practice included fasting. Two of my uncles lived there as well, completing their studies. Everyone in the house, me included, woke each day at 4:30 A.M.

Each year when the sun entered Sagittarius, my grandmother would begin a month-long practice of taking an early morning bath in the Tunga River, which flowed behind her house. It is the tradition in India to teach verses to children at a very early age—beginning with a salutation to the Eternal Teacher. On the way down to the river, she would teach me one line of a chant about the Eternal Teacher. It began, "GURU BRAHMA, GURU VIṢṆUḤU, GURU DEVO MAHEŚVARAḤA." As she chanted, I would practice my lines over and over again, looking here and there, shaking from the cold water. My grandmother would stop to listen and remind me to keep my body still, hold my spine straight, and focus on my chanting. This was how reverence for the spiritual world was introduced to my life.

Long ago in India, most people were living an ideal way of life. It did not matter whether someone was a priest, a shopkeeper, a mayor of the village, or a laborer. Each lived life in a way that led naturally to certain yogic experiences. The entire society was set up so that, based on the constitution of the individual, all members would experience yoga. This included the practice of sitting quietly each day at sunrise and sunset in order to calm the mind. This was so integrated into daily life that it was not even considered to be "practice." Rather, it was as natural as eating or sleeping.

Even fifty to one hundred years ago, people's lifestyles were far more conducive to yogic principles than they are today. In many villages there was still no electricity, and a peaceful, and quiet, lifestyle was the only option. At nighttime, the only sources of light were lanterns, candles, and fire, so people would naturally go to sleep at the optimal time. The cultural support for quieting the mind, and achieving yogic experiences, was integrated into the very fabric of life.

OUR CHALLENGE TODAY

Today, all around the globe, we have fallen into hectic, fast-paced lifestyles. Many of the exotic foods available to us keep our bodies and minds overstimulated and out of balance. Television, radio, movies, and the Internet provide us with entertainment that does not have the goal of quieting the mind; on the contrary, these entertainments are often designed to stimulate the mind. Often, this stimulation disturbs us in ways we fail to notice. As a result, we have lost something dear. Most do not even know what is missing. We are oblivious to the pervasive deterioration of our fundamental human condition.

Unlike the people of the small town where I lived with my grandmother, people now live very busy lives. They rarely, if ever, provide time to experience conditions related to the yogic journey. There are few yogis to inspire us to live differently and few examples of people living an ideal yogic way of life. We simply end up following society's trends and unconsciously pass them along to our children.

People today have lost many of the original capacities that yogis once saw present in all human beings. Like people addicted to drugs or alcohol, we have undergone a structural change in mind and body. This loss of our original condition, and its negative effects on the mind, body, and soul, is a tragedy. Because of these radical changes, even those who strive to do yogic practices may find it difficult and challenging at times. People despair that such clarity and focus are not possible in our world today. But the truth is that they are possible. Moreover, they are our birthright. And, to a large extent, that is the central theme of this book.

We have a great deal to learn about the actual impact of how we live our daily lives. The path of Aṣṭāṅga Yoga offers the practices and disciplines necessary to lead a life that is truly supportive of the highest form of human happiness. I refer to this as an *ideal* way of life, or *lifestyle.* I am also referring to the traditional definition of *Aṣṭāṅga Yoga,* rather than what has been popularized over the past several decades in the West. When we understand the connection between how we live our lives and our potential to achieve meaningful yogic experiences, we may then choose to make the necessary adjustments that can move us in the direction of *Realization* and *Liberation.*

THE PARABLE OF THE NOBLE PRINCE

Once a noble and powerful king ruled over a peaceful kingdom inhabited by honorable and worthy subjects. He dwelt in a beautiful palace with his wife and infant son. His kingdom was endowed with peace, contentment, and much material and spiritual wealth. All who lived there enjoyed a serene existence and lived in happiness.

One ill-fated day, the kingdom came under attack from a strong, malicious enemy. The king assembled his army and gathered all available resources to defend the kingdom. Though the king and his army fought valiantly, they were outnumbered and outmaneuvered. Eventually, the enemy overpowered the king's army, seriously wounded the king, and took possession of the palace and the entire kingdom.

To preserve all that was dear to them, the king's subjects helped him escape with his queen and their small son. They believed that if the king survived, so might their kingdom; if the king was killed, the kingdom would surely be lost forever.

The royal family left the palace and hid in a forest. They had no provisions, nor any means of acquiring them, and soon faced starvation. The king made every sacrifice possible for his child, feeding him all the food he could find. But one day, weak and exhausted, the king and queen died, leaving the helpless child alone. Eventually, the child crawled even deeper into the forest.

Soon afterward, a group of hunters came by chance upon the crying baby. They failed to recognize the baby as the crown prince, but they felt compassion for the small child and took him back to their village. There they fed and cared for him as one of their own. Naturally, as the boy grew, he adopted the language and traditions of his new family and the other village children. Living in a village of hunters, he, too, excelled in the skills of hunting, archery, and tracking wild game.

One day, the boy and his village companions were out hunting. In their quest, they chased game through the valleys, over hills, and through dense forests. In their enthusiastic pursuit, they lost track of their prey and became disoriented, unable to find the way back to their village. While searching for some clue to their whereabouts, they discovered a small *āśrama* in the forest. Curious, they entered and met the sage who lived there. This sage happened to be a Realized *yogi,* or *ṛṣi,* who understood the ancient science of guiding others to Realization. He possessed uncommon powers, including yogic sight, and could visualize the unseen workings of the whole universe. He was a deeply compassionate man, and everyone loved and honored him because of the guidance he offered.

This ṛṣi was a charming man who enjoyed engaging with these vibrant young hunters. He invited them to sit down and offered them delicious milk, food, and holy water. As the boys were eating and talking, the sage listened to their adventures with delight; everyone laughed until tears came to their eyes. One boy in particular caught the ṛṣi's interest. This boy was not like the other boys. Through his yogic sight, the ṛṣi recognized that this boy was not the child of a hunter but actually the son of a king.

After the boys finished eating, the ṛṣi quietly took this one boy aside and asked, "Are you from the same village as your companions?"

"Yes, sir," the boy replied. "We are all from the same village."

"And is your father from this same village?" the ṛṣi inquired.

"Yes," replied the boy. "However, he died when I was still a baby. I was raised by my uncle, whom I now regard as my father. He loves me as if I were his own son."

"And your uncle is also a hunter?" asked the ṛṣi.

"Yes, he is," said the boy.

The ṛṣi thought for a moment and then said gently, "My heart is moved to tell you something: You are not the son of a hunter, but the son of a king. Truly, you are a prince!"

This surprised the boy tremendously. "Sir, I am afraid that I don't understand. Am I somehow different from the other boys?"

"Yes," the ṛṣi answered, "there is indeed a difference."

The boy was suddenly filled with questions: "What is a prince? What are the differences between a prince and other boys? Do princes also hunt? What else does a prince do?"

As they were speaking, the other boys prepared to leave and approached the two. The ṛṣi quickly whispered to the boy, "I need to speak to you more when you have some time. Will you come visit me again?"

"Yes, sir," answered the boy. "I would like to come back."

"For now," the ṛṣi counseled him, "keep this information to yourself. Until you understand more, it would be better not to talk about this to the others in your village." He then gave the boys directions back to their village and sent them on their way home.

Honoring the ṛṣi's advice, the boy told no one about the surprising revelation. He pondered over what the holy ṛṣi had said, asking himself, "Am I not a hunter's son? How is it that I am a prince?"

Soon after, the boy returned to the āśrama, and the ṛṣi continued to explain, "A prince is the son of a kingdom's ruler. He possesses extraordinary mental and physical capacities, and a powerful and charismatic personality. He enjoys great wealth and shoulders great responsibility because the whole kingdom belongs to him. He has control over it but uses that control only for the benefit of his subjects. And though he lives in a palace, his acts are service minded, because he is always thinking of the people's welfare and of his duty as the prince of the kingdom."

The boy did not comprehend entirely, but the information had a powerful effect on his mind. As time passed, he began to feel deep love and dedication toward the ṛṣi. He returned often to the āśrama. In due course, the ṛṣi gave further explanation.

"Though you dress like the rest of the villagers, the structure of your body is different from that of theirs, as are your eyes and your smile. Your body is well proportioned and noble in stature. Your forehead is large and your chest broad. Your trunk is lean like a lion, your legs are like pillars, and your arms long and powerful. And though you speak the same language, your speech carries far more impact." The ṛṣi concluded, "These are the features of a prince."

When the boy returned to his village, he would observe small differences between the other villagers and himself. In time, he realized that these differences were quite significant. The ṛṣi continued answering his questions, explaining the duties of a prince, and imparting wisdom to him. "You are a very powerful person," the ṛṣi counseled. "Learn how to live up to your full potential."

The boy's princely qualities gradually became more and more evident with each passing day. As he gained new understanding, so grew his confidence and his ability to lead and influence others in the village. In time, he raised an army and returned to his real father's kingdom. There, he defeated his father's enemies and ascended the throne as the rightful heir.

OUR TRUE NATURE

How does this story relate to yoga? It is an allegory for the science of yoga itself. In its essence, it speaks of something at the very core of our human existence. Yoga recognizes that in this worldly kingdom, all of humanity is royalty. The Saṃskṛta word *rāja* means "king"; it is derived from the root *rajru,* meaning "light." Rāja indicates both king and the Great Light, the Eternal Truth that is the source of this universe. It is what resides at the center of each and every heart. We are incarnations of this Eternal Truth and, as such, rightful heirs to a divine kingdom. Previously, we inhabited this kingdom and lived in its splendor. But just as the prince became lost in the forest, we, too, have become lost in our worldly affairs. Just as the young prince was ignorant of his true identity, we too are ignorant of the true nature of the Self. This is because we have become overpowered by delusion and attachment to this external world, swept up in life.

Ignorance leads us to think that this life, along with its daily challenges and material rewards, is the only possible option available to us. Caught by our powerful attachments, we unknowingly have abandoned our rightful glory. Over the ages, through many births and deaths, the memory of this glorious kingdom has been buried; we have forgotten who we are and where our original kingdom resides. What is more, we have forgotten that there is even anything to remember.

OUR CAPACITY TO ENJOY SOMETHING GLORIOUS

Like the prince who lived as a hunter's child, we have adopted the lifestyle of those around us. Through the many daily activities and distractions we engage in, we have lost our connection to the glorious kingdom that was once our birthright. We once embraced an ideal way of life but now have discarded and forgotten what it means to live in such a way. Since we are no longer able to recollect these original experiences, we have given up the ideal way of life that supports them.

Moreover, not only have we forgotten who we truly are, we have developed highly injurious misconceptions and habits that rob us of our original inherent powers. Like the prince in the story, we have lost our capacity for enjoying something glorious, a natural bliss that would continuously fill our hearts if we were living in our original state. Having returned to the palace, the prince once again experienced power, glory, and his divine qualities. If we return to a pure and sound human mind and body, we, too, will be able to experience the magnificence and divinity of our original Self.

But how do we regain the capacity to experience such things? How can we see who we truly are? As children of the Eternal Truth, it is our right to experience the Eternal Truth in our daily lives and to enjoy the unsurpassed pleasure it brings. But to achieve this we need to be reminded of who we are. How is this possible? Who and what can help us achieve this?

THE SCIENCE OF YOGA

Yoga is a systematic and scientific method for awakening the memory of our original state. A proper yoga teacher knows how to remind the student who he or she truly is and how to stimulate and bring forth the student's forgotten capacities. As a first step, the teacher catches the heart of the student and kindles the flame of desire for spiritual happiness. Then the teacher tames the student's mind, so the intellect becomes an able and willing partner in the journey toward Realization. A teacher who is able to do this is an authentic teacher. This kind of teaching is only possible when it is derived from the teacher's direct experience. When it comes from his heart, it can carry divine messages directly to the heart of the student. Only a person with sight can lead the blind; only one who has achieved Self-Realization can guide others to Enlightenment. Such a Realized being is the *guru,* or the *Eternal Teacher.*

A Realized person should remind us that we are not meant for suffering. Is suffering natural and intrinsic to our experience? Does some Divine entity bestow unhappiness upon us, and are we powerless to refuse it? Certainly not. We have created our own misery; we also have the capacity to eliminate it. It is not necessary to be unhappy. We have the right and capacity to live in a wonderful world filled with experiences of bliss. What keeps us from doing so? It is only our ignorance about who we are and where we have come from.

Education under a Realized person will enlighten us about ourselves. Gradually, we will be able to recognize our present condition and learn about our great internal capacity. His teachings will purify us, and we will gain insight into our own souls. We will see that we are the Eternal Truth and that our lost kingdom is to be found not outside ourselves, but within. In this way, we will restore our body and mind to their original states. We will come to understand that although we are living in this external world, this is not our permanent place; we are merely visitors. Our permanent abode is inside. In fact, this Eternal Truth is the source of all life and the entire Universe. It is the ultimate goal, a final destination we arrive at through Realization and a place where we may remain forever.

For thousands of years, the great sages have sought to fully understand how Realization occurs. Yogis have identified many aspects of the mind and body that work to support the yogic experience. A comprehensive yogic science has emerged that recognizes the uniqueness of the human mind and body. If properly working, the mind and body enable humans to directly experience the Eternal Truth. This experience, as well as the bliss that ensues, is amazing. This unique capacity available to human beings helps us confirm that the very goal of human life is to experience yoga.

THE FOURTH STATE

The Indian science of traditional medicine called Āyurveda uses the word *svastha* to describe a healthy person. In Saṃskṛta, *sva* means "the

Soul." One who operates in this external world at the behest of the Soul is svastha. A svastha realizes the Truth and lives according to that Realization. In all the ancient Indian sciences, the idea of health directly or indirectly implies the existence of the yogic experience. It is the experience of countless yogis that demonstrates just how natural, and extraordinary, the yogic condition is.

Of the conditions that we experience in our daily lives, we are most aware of the *waking state*. We engage in various activities, including working, eating, moving from place to place, and conversing with others. Then, at the end of the day, we go home and at some point, go to sleep. At first, while falling asleep, we will experience a few minutes of *dreaming*. We see images in our minds, some of which make sense, and some of which may make no sense at all. Then the mind, in need of complete relaxation, transitions to *deep sleep*. While in this state, we have neither dreams nor consciousness of the external world. We may stay in this state for a period of time. After sleeping deeply for some time, we start to dream again. After dreaming, again we will fall back into a deep sleep. This pattern is repeated throughout the night until we arise in the morning.

These three natural states of being—*waking, dreaming,* and *deep sleep*—occur in other animals, as well as human beings. These are natural states and usually require little or no training. However, for human beings alone, there is a most important natural *fourth* state; it is the state of *Samādhi, yoga,* or *sahajāvasthā*. The word *sahaja* means "endowed by birth"; *avasthā* means "state." Just as the ṛṣi reminded the prince of his natural abilities, this fourth state of mind is natural, but it is present only when there is total balance and health in body and mind. Once a yoga practitioner has significantly balanced his or her body and mind, and becomes firmly established in the experience of Samādhi, he or she will begin to notice the daily cycle of these states.

SAMĀDHI

Today's definition of health is not comprehensive; unfortunately, many important qualities and ideas are left out. This is because most people acknowledge only three states of existence for the mind and fail to recognize this all-important fourth state.

If we are living balanced lives, we will automatically wake up at a certain time in the morning without the need of an alarm clock. At midday we will feel energized and motivated to work hard. Our appetite will arise at particular times throughout the day. We will feel sleepy at night and fall asleep without a struggle.

For the most part, our society recognizes our profound need for sleep, as well as the negative impact on our health if we lose the capacity to sleep. If there were a society that had developed the capacity to exist without sleep, its definition of health would not include good sleep.

Using this analogy, we might ask, Why do people lose the capacity to sleep? Some people might consume unsuitable food or worry too much. Some might crave material objects and work too hard in their effort to acquire them. Perhaps they have mental strain from a frantic lifestyle. They might simply stay up too late and not follow their natural sleep pattern. Most often, it is an unhealthy lifestyle that disrupts people's sleep.

This is the same with the experience of the fourth state, or Samādhi. If our lives are in total health and balance, Samādhi will naturally occur regularly at a particular hour of the day. At such a time, the mind will start feeling a particular type of happiness and a separation from the external world. This feeling compels the yogi to find a private, quiet place to sit and meditate. Just as sleepiness is a sign to indicate that we need sleep, the practitioner's craving for bliss is the sign that the conditions for Samādhi are available. If the practitioner heeds this message and sits in a calm and quiet place, he may reach this wonderful experience of Samādhi.

However, most of us are not around people who go into Samādhi regularly. Thus, we do not consider it as natural as sleeping or eating. Many believe that Samādhi is something novel to achieve through great and meticulous effort. That is in one way a mistaken idea.

The absence of the yogic condition is due to a wide variety of errors in our way of living today. Because these errors have been perpetuated over many generations, we have developed ignorance about the naturalness and even necessity of yogic experiences. Most have forgotten about the very existence of the yogic state and accept that its absence is natural. We understand little about what constitutes an ideal way of life and its benefits. Nor do we grasp the mechanics of the yogic condition, or understand the relationship between lifestyle and Samādhi. This loss of understanding about our true nature is a form of blindness.

KALI YUGA

We are living in the *Kali Yuga,* a vast cycle of time within the evolution of the universe. It is characterized by its drastic changes and turmoil. According to the ancient ṛṣis, this is an age in which human beings develop to be highly extroverted and thus lose their capacity for inward awareness of the Self. Though conditions are challenging for Enlightenment, one should remain optimistic and strive to develop a yogic lifestyle. Though an aspirant may not have the benefit of a Realized teacher, one should continue to seek and experiment on one's own. This too may be considered a path toward Enlightenment. There are indicators and reminders everywhere—but only for a serious and true aspirant. There are many stories throughout history of yogis who became Realized even though they lacked prior training, guidance, or the use of any yogic practices. The human system naturally possesses the capacity to experience yoga. But in order to access that capacity, we must have clear intentions.

OUR ULTIMATE GOAL

The culmination of yoga is Realization, which arrives through the experience of Samādhi. Each healthy human being should experience Samādhi. This central idea provides the context for us to explore the vast subject of yoga. With this purpose, we begin to understand why the sages recommend various disciplines and explain the impact those practices have on reaching this goal. Through the study of yoga, we can comprehend how the body and mind enable the yogic experience to manifest. If we are able to follow these yogic disciplines, we will maintain the health of this body and mind. In this way, our human effort will have maximum impact in this life—not simply for ourselves, but also for the benefit of others. We need not accept these ideas on faith alone; rather, we should test and validate them for ourselves.

Like the young prince who sought the benevolent ṛṣi's advice to understand his true nature and where he had come from, we, too, must make a sincere effort to understand our full capacity as human beings. Then we, too, will discover who we truly are and recollect the Eternal Truth.

CHAPTER TWO

THE BLISS OF SAMĀDHI

आनन्दः

THE MOST IMPORTANT benefit of experiencing the Eternal Truth is the state of bliss that it brings. This bliss is what all human beings unconsciously crave. Most people who would read a book about yoga may no longer try to obtain happiness through such misguided means as alcohol, drugs, promiscuous sex, and the like. However, we do many other things that we think will bring the happiness we crave. We may seek more money, better relationships, a job promotion, a fit body, or a vacation. Some of us have grown more sophisticated and strive after less tangible goals such as education, prestige, or successful children. None of these pursuits are bad in and of themselves. But when we expect them to bring true happiness, we will likely pursue them in an imbalanced fashion. In the end, we will most likely be left disappointed and unfulfilled.

For example, some may think that acquisition of wealth and its many material advantages will bring happiness. This is a delusion. Such people reach for money everywhere and in the process sacrifice other important elements of life. They often find themselves in conflict with those around them and create harmful competition in society. At its extreme, grasping for wealth causes much pain, grief, and chaos.

Until an aspirant knows the bliss of the Eternal Truth achieved through the yogic experience of Samādhi, her craving for happiness will remain insatiable. Because of her desperate, never-ending search for this elusive prize, she will continue to engage in inappropriate activities that never bring the reward she craves. Once she experiences yogic happiness, all these unwanted activities will come to an end. It is not that she will stop participating in the external world; rather, the context from which she operates will change. She will approach all activities with yogic happiness in mind. Above all else, she will be careful not to disrupt this state. It is this new point of reference that leads an aspirant to correct thoughts and actions in all areas of life.

WORLDLY HAPPINESS

The difference between divine bliss and the happiness we find in the world is that the latter is based on an external cause. When we use or consume objects, we often feel a measure of happiness. This feeling appears when we acquire a particular material or fulfill a particular desire, but it vanishes sooner or later. It is transitory. Even though we have the object of our desire directly in front of us, we will not always feel the expected elation.

For example, the first time we purchase a new car we feel a great deal of pleasure. We enjoy the car completely—its new smell, its clean interior, and so on. Later, as the car ages, we do not enjoy it as much. The next time we purchase a new car we may feel happy again but not as happy as the first time.

Food is another example. Many people use food to make themselves happy. They may even describe an experience with certain foods as providing a kind of "bliss." Companies who market foods have readily capitalized on this phenomenon by promising such experiences. But the experience is only temporary. The body eventually becomes full and satisfied. If too much of one food or another is eaten, the body will begin to reject it and even find it repulsive.

This is the nature of worldly happiness. It is transient and dependent upon worldly materials. Yet even the availability of materials does not ensure that we will feel happy or content. Instead of realizing the nature of this transient happiness, we automatically switch our desire to some new object or material and repeat the process. We crave the new material, seek it, acquire it, feel happy for a short time, become bored with it, and no longer feel happy. This kind of enjoyment may even do injury to our mind and body. Though some people feel a lot of gratification eating sweets or fatty foods, for example, over time that food may damage their health.

Worldly happiness does have a relationship to yogic happiness. When we acquire a new material, or achieve a worldly goal, we temporarily feel completely satisfied. For a time, there is no desire and fewer thoughts. The feeling of contentment is actually caused by the temporary cessation of desires and thoughts. The door of internal pleasure is opened slightly, and a small trace of internal happiness peers through our heart. This is the true source of the pleasure we feel; thus, the happiness is only indirectly related to the new material or achievement. While we may find some satisfaction by acquiring more and more worldly materials, that is only an apparent source of our happiness. The endless pursuit of these materials will lead to imbalance within our systems and ultimately sickness. It is much wiser to find our happiness directly by learning to reduce our desires and calm our mind. This is the surest path to lasting contentment.

The happiness derived from the yogic experience is internal and independent, its source eternal. It does not originate from any object. It comes from nothing, "no thing." It does not occur for any reason—and therein lies its greatness. Nor does such happiness cause any type of side effect or harm to our body. On the contrary, it rectifies the body and mind. And because it comes from inside, one cannot exhaust it. An aspirant will not become tired of this joy, or fear that he might lose it, unlike the happiness that comes from the purchase of a new computer or smartphone. Nor will he develop any kind of aversion to the source of the happiness, as we do when we eat too much delicious food. It is like a flood, flowing downward from the top of the body. And after an aspirant becomes established in this experience, he may even come to enjoy this bliss in his waking state. Once this bliss starts flowing, it is experienced twenty-four hours a day, bringing wonderful balance to our entire system.

Of course, we need not entirely avoid the experience of happiness that comes from acquiring materials. Like divine happiness, worldly materials are also offered through the grace of Nature. When a healthy, balanced person eats good food, he feels happy. Worldly happiness is not bad; this body is meant for both yoga and *bhoga,* or the enjoyment of material and sensory experience of this world. But worldly pleasures should not disturb an aspirant's system and prevent him from enjoying divine bliss. All pleasures should be in accordance with the principles of yoga and ultimately support our mind and body to experience divine happiness.

A BOAT TO SAIL THIS WORLDLY OCEAN

In order for this divine communication to occur, we must understand the degree to which the material world impacts our life. Each object has its purpose, and its essential nature determines its use. For this reason, we need to carefully consider the characteristics and properties of an object. Though we may intend to use something correctly, we often do not understand its best use. This misunderstanding results in our misuse of many objects and materials. We should think about the appropriate use of worldly materials and not use anything in a haphazard way.

For instance, we make decisions about the use of a tree based on the tree's innate properties, as well as our needs. What benefits will it provide us? What is its most important benefit? We can swing on a rope hung from a branch, relax in its shade, or harvest its lumber for building houses or furniture. However, if it is a fruit-bearing tree, we will value it differently. We will not cut it down just for wood, but treasure it for its fruit. We may enjoy its shade and, when the tree dies, use its wood, but these are secondary benefits compared to what is most important—delicious fruit.

Likewise, light is used for many purposes. In Las Vegas, casinos use millions of light bulbs to keep gamblers up for the entire night. Is this a proper use of light? In this light they misuse their minds, bodies, and money. Alternatively, we can use light to see what fully supports the health of our mind and body. We can even meditate on light, which may remind us of our original Self.

Throughout the ages, sages have used yogic sight to determine how best to use food, air, water, animals, plants, rocks, and minerals—in short, everything in this universe—with the intention of discovering how it helps or hinders yoga practice. If a yogi wants to learn about an object or material, he will use certain yogic techniques to focus his mind. This inward movement of the mind becomes a compass that guides the wise to know the proper use of materials. Many striking and invaluable insights about the nature and use of materials result from these techniques. A scientist, scholar, artist, or common man may be using aspects of these yogic techniques when he or she engages in deep contemplation on a particular matter. Most of these shared techniques involve disciplining the mind to focus on a single object, problem, or thought, while limiting other distractions. This kind of deep contemplation is also a type of Samādhi—though a lower, initial form of Samādhi.

Even our human body, mind, and five senses are considered "materials" of this world. We use these as tools to make our way through this life. Moreover, they are the most important materials and the ones closest to us. They are wonderful, complex instruments, like the instruments of a boat with which we can sail this worldly ocean.

USE OF MIND, BODY, AND SENSES

We may use the mind to delve into the sciences of the universe or to play games for entertainment and competition. Or we can use the mind to devise plots and cause trouble to those around us. We can use the human body for hard work, fun, and enjoyment, or to physically attack someone. In the same way, we can use our senses to examine the properties of materials around us or simply for entertainment, like watching movies or playing games. We might even cause serious damage to ourselves, and others, when the use of our senses leads to addiction.

But have we discovered the best possible use of our mind, body, and senses? Yogis who have pondered this question have found that the astonishing experience of Samādhi is possible through these natural gifts. Through this experience, we regain our own lost kingdom. Like the prince in the story, we discover who we truly are. Through such experiences, we enjoy a bliss that is incomparable to any other.

When the mind moves toward the experience of the Eternal Truth, that is yoga. When it migrates in the direction of the external world, that is bhoga. Yogic philosophy never rejects the material world or the enjoyment of the senses and sensory objects. It simply recommends that they be used correctly and meaningfully. The primary purpose of the mind and body is to experience yoga; its secondary purpose is to experience bhoga. Therefore, our interactions with this external world should not conflict with yoga; rather, they should fully support it. A wise person uses his mind, body, and senses primarily for the purpose of yoga; to do otherwise is to squander them.

THE INTERNAL AND EXTERNAL

Normally our mind is almost entirely associated with the external world. The poet William Wordsworth made this point when he wrote, "The world is too much with us." When our mind leaves the connection with the external world and moves internally, it will enjoy something priceless in connection with the Self. This itself is yoga.

The purpose of all yoga practices is to pave the way for moving internally to discover the Eternal Truth, to experience it, and to bring its bliss back to the mind level, sense level, and body level. This is possible only if the mind and body are working properly.

In ancient days, there was a practice to appoint a minister who served as liaison between the king and his subjects. He interacted with the public, understood their problems, and relayed matters back to the king. He might visit a village and discover the need for a canal to supply water to a fertile area of land. He would consult with the king, then inform the public about a proposed public works and schedule the work to be done. In this way, the minister conveyed messages from the public to the king, the king to the public, and the public's response back to the king.

Analogously, the king represents the Eternal Truth, the public symbolizes the body and five senses, and the mind acts as the minister in a healthy individual. As the minister moves in two directions, so should the mind. Problems we grapple with externally may be carried inwardly to the Eternal Truth through the mind. Using the support of the Eternal Truth, the inner mind can discover solutions to any dilemma and carry those solutions back to the external world. The most important message that the mind carries back from the Eternal Truth concerns the bliss and happiness that originate there. This bliss is by far the most powerful antidote to any problem. The mind's duty is to bring it back to the body and senses. This bliss develops harmony, not only within the individual, but also within the family and the whole of society.

Because the senses of most human beings are overengaged, the mind tends to linger in the external. Returning to the analogy: We have forgotten the king, the Eternal Truth. The mind no longer goes inside to retrieve the message from the Eternal Truth and carry it to the surface of the sensory level. It is as if the minister had usurped power from the king and was creating havoc by not consulting him.

Experiences in the external world of bhoga can support one's yogic path. If these experiences are in harmony with the Eternal Truth, they can lead toward Realization. This works when one surrenders the pleasures of the world to the Divine, or Supreme Being. It is also a matter of acknowledging that all activities, as well as the fruit of those activities, arise from the Divine. Even eating some delicious food may lead to yogic conditions, providing that particular pleasure is surrendered properly.

In this way, the mind has the capacity to carry the joys of the external world inward. When we experience some splendor in this external world such as a beautiful flower, a still lake, or a lovely rain shower, our enjoyment supports the mind to experience a small taste of the Eternal Truth and thus advances our yoga path. The purpose of all yoga practices is to move toward the Eternal Truth, experience it, and bring the bliss back to the mind level, sense level, and body level.

NATURE AS TEACHER

The great sage Patañjali, who was considered an authority on yogic science, affirmed in the Yoga Sūtras that yoga is natural. The first aphorism of Patañjali's Yoga Sūtras says, "*Atha yoga anuśāsanam.*" In Saṃskṛta, *śāsanam* means "commandment." The prefix *anu* means it is a commandment given by another, in this case by the Divine, Nature, or God. The full meaning here is that Patañjali is simply a messenger of the Divine, or Nature, and not the originator of these ideas.

Analogously, gravity is a dimension of nature that Sir Isaac Newton understood and described as the law of gravity. Of course, Newton did not state that he created this law; he stated that it was a *Law of Nature*; he was only a messenger who discovered and wrote it down.

If a human being issues a command, the authority of that person determines whether it should be followed or not. However, Nature is totally impartial; its authority is immutable and unchangeable, and we will not escape the consequences of its laws. Day will be followed by night, and life will be followed by death. Therefore, it is our duty to honor Nature's Laws.

What we experience as unrest in the modern lifestyle is deeply connected to our ignoring Nature's Laws. Though we have the ingrained habit of living without Samādhi, this loss has caused many radically adverse changes in our body. Each healthy human being should experience Samādhi. Despite changes in our body and mind, it is still possible to recognize some of the signs of yogic experiences occurring naturally in our lives.

RECOGNIZING THE YOGIC EXPERIENCE

According to the Upaniṣads, the traditional scriptures of India, during the eighth month of pregnancy, the fetus will experience the Eternal Truth. Because of this, at the time of birth, the child's Soul, or *jīva,* offers a prayer to God that she will remember this sacred experience, even though she is receiving a human birth. Immediately after the baby is born, she cries due to having lost that experience. Nonetheless, for the first few weeks, she will remain connected to the divine and spiritual world.

During this time, the infant may at times experience unprovoked delight. For instance, she might display a very sweet, contented smile. At other times, for no apparent reason and with no external stimulus, she might start a very innocent, pleasant kind of laughter that has an entirely different quality from the laughter of an older child. Her eyes might move upwards to the third eye and remain transfixed for some time. In such a case, there will be an appearance of freshness in her face, along with noticeable signs of contentment, happiness, and pleasure. In this state, she will not be interested in material objects, nor will she have much sensory perception; in particular, she will have little sensation of touch. At this point, the baby's pulse rate may even be reduced. Her eyes will be very clear, the iris and pupil dark and shiny; the whites will be very bright, and there will be a slight reddish tint at the outer edges. In some cases, the baby's hands and fingers will form particular shapes, positions, or *mudrās.* These signs indicate that the baby is experiencing a pure, unconditioned state. She is showing us a glimpse of the yogic experience, Samādhi.

These same signs can also be observed in an advanced yoga practitioner. As a yogi enters into Samādhi, we may see him laugh or smile for no apparent reason. We may notice a look of happiness, contentment, and pleasure in his face. His eyes will look upward naturally. He will have no sensation or external feeling, and his pulse rate will decrease. Even if he opens his eyes, he will not see anything in the external world. His skin will look shiny. The appearance of his eyes will be similar or identical to what has been described for the baby, and his hands may display the same mudrās.

The baby's experience is not as vivid as the yogi's, nor does it continue over time. As the baby grows, her mind will gradually become clouded. She will forget the unconditioned state she experienced in the first month of life. This new conditioning of her mind is due to *māyā,* screens of ignorance that begin to cover the mind. In order for *karma* and *saṃskāra* from previous births to take effect, Nature covers the mind through the help of māyā. If the baby were to fully remember the period prior to māyā's influence, she would grow up as a Realized being.

Unfortunately, because of the extroverted nature of our society, we try to attract babies to the external world. We shake toys in front of them to grab their attention. We play with them in order to provoke their lively response. By the time babies can talk, the memory of their yogic experiences will have long disappeared. Wise parents might refrain from provoking extroverted behavior in these early days, weeks, and even years. Instead, they ought to encourage their child's natural, introverted nature.

We are all born with curiosity about the world we live in. As we grow, this curiosity may evolve into a particular interest. Our interest might lean toward the beauty of science, mathematics, history, or the arts. If we probe a subject deeply with our mind, we may find ourselves naturally seeking a quiet place to sit comfortably. We may even close our eyes to better focus our attention, or we might stare into space. We will mentally block out all sounds and lose awareness of our surroundings. Even if someone calls us, we will not hear. As we concentrate deeply, and if we observe closely, we may notice changes in our breathing. Gradually, the speed of our breath will decrease, and at the point where the mind fully engages with our subject, the breath may even stop for a little while. At this exact point, we might comprehend an important aspect about our subject and feel very happy. According to yoga, this is actually a kind of transcendental state, or lower level of Samādhi itself, and it occurs naturally without any special effort on our part.

There are other common human experiences that relate to the yogic experience. For example, we might feel very happy without understanding the reason. At the peak of this experience, we might even experience breathlessness. We might assume a specific posture, see a bright light, or hear a particular sound. We might even have a feeling of losing consciousness. Our body might exhibit a particular kind of relaxation and our skin become smooth, with a pleasant color. These phenomena are not necessarily due to some yoga technique; they occur naturally but can be identified by those who recognize their significance. These, too, are lower levels of Samādhi.

EXPERIENCING THE SELF

The experience of the Eternal Truth eliminates ignorance and changes the aspirant dramatically in many ways. The spark of this Great Light within us is itself known as the Soul. It is who we are. But sadly, we are mostly oblivious to it. When the Soul is experienced through Samādhi, one suddenly understands who she truly is. With this understanding, she will be naturally drawn to engage in activities that are in alignment with her own true nature. She will cease meaningless endeavors that develop more karma and saṃskāra. Self-Realization brings absolute clarity. It is the door for Liberation. There is no other way out of human bondage.

Once a person has Realized the Self, she is Liberated for the rest of her life, even though she still possesses a body. Though she still carries the karmas and saṃskāras of her previous births—and must experience their consequences—she will no longer be attached in any way to her actions. She will live like everyone else—waking, sleeping, eating, and breathing. The great difference is that she regularly experiences the Self. A flood of bliss pervades her life. She never forgets who she really is. Because of her detached mentality, her actions will no longer cause further bondage.

Because of the flood of bliss that saturates her life, the Self-Realized person does not have any desires for further human experiences. All other experience pales beside her experience of Samādhi.

When a child discovers more complex toys, he will quit playing with alphabet blocks. In a similar way, one who is Liberated will not have much interest in worldly desires; the internal world is incomparably more attractive. Because she is free of all desires, all further actions of this birth will be performed as her duty, free from attachment. Like fried seeds that will not grow, accumulated karma of previous births will have lost its power. Hence, when she leaves her body, she will not be reborn. Her individual Soul will be united with the Universal Soul, the Eternal Truth. This is the final Liberation.

CHAPTER THREE

THE PATH TO REALIZATION

मोक्षमार्गः

THE TALLEST MOUNTAIN in the world, Mount Everest, known in Saṃskṛta as *Gaurishankara,* can be seen from many different places. It can be seen from great distances and even from several different countries. Different locations and points of view offer entirely different perspectives of the same mountain. Yet, regardless of one's vantage point, the mountain remains the same.

Likewise, yoga is one of six basic Indian philosophies that offer various vantage points, or *darśanas,* from which to view our lives. Even though these darśanas vary in their perspective, the object of their inquiry and focus remains the same—Realization of the Eternal Truth.

What if we wish to actually climb the mountain and reach its summit? One path may gradually wind its way through forests and gentle inclines; another may go steeply up rocks and cliffs. The experience of climbing the mountain will vary according to the path one chooses. This will also influence one's point of view of the mountain. Nevertheless, each path will lead to the same destination—the mountain's glorious summit.

In a similar way, it is a combination of one's darśana, or vision, and one's individual yogic path that will determine one's course and one's experience in reaching the final goal. This is partly why there are so many varied definitions of yoga and ways to describe the yogic journey. Though the definitions vary, they all lead the practitioner to the same ultimate experience of the Great Light.

THE NATURE OF MIND

Because the mind is one of the primary tools used to reach this final goal, it is essential to learn how it works. Throughout the ages, yogis have gained significant insight into the mechanism of the mind. In the Yoga Sūtras, Patañjali defines yoga as "*Yogaścitta vṛtti nirodhaḥ.*" This may be translated as "Yoga is the restraint of the modifications of mind." In its natural state, the mind is like a leaf blown by the wind; it constantly moves from place to place. This is what is meant by the word *modifications*, or as Patañjali says, *vṛtti*. In Saṃskṛta, the closest literal translation for this word is "existence." Thus, the mind's existence itself can be grasped in the form of constant change, or continual modification. We might also think of vṛtti as vibrations, or waves of the mind. Just as a cloud changes shape, though remains a cloud, so too does the mind change yet remain the mind.

Furthermore, Patañjali says that all these modifications of the mind fit into one of five categories: right knowledge, wrong knowledge, imagination, sleep, and memory. There are many thousands of modifications of the mind, but all fit into one of these five categories. By taking an analytical approach, we can observe the mind's various activities and learn how they fit into these categories.

Our mind receives sensory input from our senses of sight, smell, taste, touch, and hearing. If our senses are in good health, and external conditions support their proper functioning, then information that we receive from them will be correct. In fact, the quality of our daily life often depends on receiving correct information from our senses. We see a white liquid, and because it has a certain smell and taste, we conclude that it is milk. We eat fruits and vegetables, such as carrots, apples, oranges, and mangos, and assess that they are good for our health. At times we crosscheck our conclusions with others to confirm our assessment. These are examples of right knowledge, or *pramāṇa*. They are modifications of the mind derived from various types of sensory observation, right inference, and trustworthy testimonials.

However, the mind does not always receive information correctly. If we are walking along a dark path at night and see a coiled rope, we might confuse it with a snake. Or we might meet a man on a train and think he'd make a good friend. Later, we might learn that we misread him and that we have met no friend at all. Many people who have spent hours in the sun getting deep, rich tans later develop skin cancer and regret having believed that so much exposure was a good thing. Perhaps a young person believes that drinking alcohol is harmless fun.

Later, if he studies the effects of alcohol on the mind, as well as its effects on meditation, he will realize he was wrong. Prior to realizing our error, such modifications of the mind are known as wrong knowledge, or delusion, which in Saṃskṛta is *viparyaya.* Wrong knowledge is due to incorrect sensory input, faulty reasoning, or false testimonials.

We generally have very active imaginations. We can visualize what the future may bring or what the past might have brought, had it unfolded differently. We can even visualize things abstractly—things that have no basis in past, present, or future reality. In the Yoga Sūtras, Patañjali calls this type of modification *vikalpa,* which may be translated as "imagination." For example, we can think of a golden lotus flower floating in the sky. No example of this can be found in the world; it is a purely imaginary idea.

The fourth modification of the mind is sleep, or *nidrā.* After any stress or strain, the mind needs to relax. When our day is finished, we go to sleep. Next to the yogic experience, sleep brings the greatest degree of relaxation and benefit to the mind.

The fifth modification of the mind Patañjali refers to is memory, or *smṛti*—specifically, memory of the previous four modifications we have already mentioned. We have the ability to remember our previous day and the right knowledge we experienced on that day. We can also recall what we have imagined and whether our sleep was restful. While this is related to the first four, it operates in a way that is distinct from them. It allows us to recollect the others and is itself known as memory.

All modifications of the mind fit into one of these five categories that Patañjali has outlined. Even human emotions are based on these five modifications. Yet is this the full nature of the mind? No. Even though our most familiar experience is for the mind to move and wander, it also has the capacity to remain still and calm. When practicing yoga, our main intention is to reduce these modifications of the mind and encourage this stillness. Once all mental activity ceases, what remains is a profound deep silence. To define yoga as the restraint of the mind's modifications is another way of indicating the state of Samādhi.

Our mind is often fixed on the external world. We see a sunset, hear music, smell flowers, feel a cool breeze, reminisce over days past, and plan for our future. Our mind is like a screen where something is always being projected, always making an impression. The more we fill our minds with external objects, the more we are entangled in the external world. However, if we stop these external engagements using a spiritual intention, we will be able to recognize the Great Light, the Eternal Truth, as it is projected on the mind.

Although this Great Light is ever present, we are not aware of it, because we focus on external objects. Since our interest is elsewhere, the Eternal Truth is obscured. When the mind withdraws from worldly objects, it gradually begins to recognize this light. Further, as the experience of this light expands to the fullest extent, a practitioner's enjoyment increases proportionately. The mind will dissolve into the light and lose the illusion of being separate. It will merge into its original condition, or *causal state, pradhāna.*

FOUR TOOLS: FOUR STATES OF THE MIND

In the West, the concept of *mind* generally refers to the thinking instrument that develops external thoughts and ideas. As such, the mind is constantly changing, shifting from one thought to the next. In yogic theory, the concept of the mind is simultaneously more specific and more comprehensive.

In yoga, the mind is understood to operate in four distinct ways, or *states.* These are sometimes referred to as the *four tools.* They are named *pradhāna, mahat, ahaṅkāra,* and *manas.* These are important concepts for an aspirant to grasp. There are no equivalent English words, but they can be understood through close study and by observing how our own mind functions.

The first thing to understand is that yoga involves a reverse process of evolution, or *de-evolution.* It is a process of the mind moving from the external world to its original condition, or causal state. It describes the mind moving inward. Let us clarify a few terms that are vital to understanding this process.

In our waking state, *manas* is the part of the mind that we experience most of the time. It is what we normally refer to in English when speaking of the mind. In this condition of mind we are watching a parade of external objects. As we leave for work, we search for our keys and pocketbook. We walk out the door and lock it. We greet the neighbor as we walk down the street to the bus. We board the bus and pay the fare. Manas is the tool we use to apprehend external objects, one after another. Just as a monkey hops from branch to branch in a tree, so manas continuously wanders from place to place.

Ahaṅkāra is a state of mind that maintains a consciousness of "I." We all have some familiarity with this aspect of the mind. Sometimes we are completely absorbed in external objects; at other times, while thinking, walking, or looking into a mirror, we feel a consciousness of "I." The external object is there, and so is the "I." But if we focus our mind and come to a state where the "I" is constant rather than intermittent, then manas fully merges into ahaṅkāra. In the state of ahaṅkāra, the mind operates like a lens through which one views pure "I" consciousness.

We can learn to recognize a third state of mind through a type of happiness that comes to us for no apparent reason. This is the *mahat* state, sometimes referred to as *buddhi* or *citta*. Though this bliss is always present to some degree, we rarely recognize it, because we are preoccupied with the external world. But we may get small tastes of it from time to time in our daily activities. For example, perhaps we have been engaged in some research and after making a discovery, we get a deep feeling of satisfaction. This is evidence of the mind linked to mahat. On the yogic journey, the mind has the capacity to become fully absorbed in this kind of happiness. In such moments, the mind rests in mahat.

The fourth and final state is *pradhāna,* where the mind becomes totally still. Pradhāna is the state of Realization.

These are the four distinct ways the mind functions. Each state emerges through a de-evolutionary process as the mind moves inward, returning to its original causal state. As manas returns to its causal state, it merges into ahaṅkāra, where the consciousness of "I" resides. Ahaṅkāra itself merges into mahat, where one experiences a bliss unassociated with the external world. Finally, mahat merges into pradhāna, where the mind becomes completely still and Realization occurs.

Conversely, the opposite process brings the mind from its causal state back to the external world: the previously described order being reversed. Beginning with pradhāna, the source, the mind moves to mahat, then to ahaṅkāra, and finally to manas, where it becomes totally immersed in the external world once again. In this process, manas is caused by ahaṅkāra, which itself is caused by mahat, which is caused by pradhāna.

Prior to Realization, the bliss or happiness one experiences in the mahat state is not an emotion; it is something entirely different. Emotions are related to external objects, combined with some preconditioning. Without this preconditioning, a practitioner would view all objects and materials with natural equanimity. Lacking attachment or aversion, he would experience everything—success and failure, pain and pleasure—evenly and with a calm and steady mind. When happiness is associated with an object, it carries emotional attachments linked with this preconditioning.

If we focus the mind on something, its ability to grasp the object of our focus expands. Conversely, if we ignore the same object, the mind's power to grasp it is reduced. This is the nature of the mind. Our mental faculties function like muscles. Without regular exercise, both will atrophy. After a long break from her studies, a mathematician will often find that it takes some time before she regains her former sharpness and abilities. This should not be confused with simply giving the external focus of the mind some rest. There are famous examples of scientists and mathematicians who have had sudden and profound understanding of a problem after momentarily shifting their focus elsewhere. In these cases, it is manas that has shifted its focus, while the fully engaged mahat is responsible for solving the problem.

Mahat may seem like a difficult state to achieve, but this is mostly because one has not consistently focused on it. Simple lack of experience has limited the mind's ability to reach it. But if one reflects deeply upon mahat, the mind will begin to automatically merge with it. This experience will expand until ahaṅkāra dissolves into mahat, so only mahat exists. Even though the resultant bliss may seem unreachable, through dedicated practice one can attain it.

MEMORY AS A YOGIC TOOL

Remembering—and even memorizing—happiness is a fundamental skill in yoga. A proper yoga practice will naturally bring happiness and joy. Each day, during his practice, a student should recall any thread of happiness or joy that may have previously been experienced while practicing. By doing this, a practitioner will develop a unique skill, and progress on the yogic path will accelerate. Unfortunately, there is a trend in today's world to memorize worries. Some people will even search for something to worry about and obsess upon it. This is a kind of torture to the mind that robs it of the happiness and joy we crave.

YOGA AS SAMĀDHI

The mind has both the capacity to move and jump like a flame in the open air and the capacity to be extremely still like a protected flame. When practitioners notice they are experiencing fewer thoughts, they are approaching the mahat state. If they use these quiet times well, they will eventually arrive at a condition of total calm. This is pradhāna. In pradhāna, one finds supreme quietness or stillness, like a lamp in a windless cave. If there are no objects in the mind, it will be absolutely still.

Pradhāna is that which has no modifications and possesses total stillness. Just as birds leave their nests each morning in search of food, then return again in the evening, so the mind will return to its causal state, its source: pradhāna. Some yogis also explain this as Samādhi. Understanding this mechanism through their yogic experience, these yogis define yoga itself as Samādhi.

WITHDRAWAL OF THE FIVE SENSES

Some people feel the need to be doing something all the time. For them, sitting motionless for a little while may seem like a waste of time. Learning to find the quietness in the mind is not an easy task, but it is rewarding. From time to time, everyone will unconsciously come upon some aspects of the yogic experience. We might find ourselves in a beautiful place in nature and suddenly feel the urge to sit down and let our mind be quiet. Or we might be working hard on a project and suddenly realize that we have been sitting motionless, staring off into space. This is by the grace of Nature, and is to be cherished. It is a kind of yogic experience.

If five running horses are pulling a chariot, it is possible to control that chariot only by controlling the horses. Our mind, the driver of the chariot, holds the reins to these horses, which represent our five senses. If our mind wants to slow down or stop, it must learn to control the five senses until it is able to withdraw them completely. Having understood this while in Samādhi, some great yogis define yoga as controlling the five senses to the fullest extent.

EXPERIENCE OF "I" ITSELF

As we have said in our description of ahaṅkāra, our awareness of "I" is a reflection of the Eternal Truth filtered through the modifications of the mind. As we explore the realms of the mind, and closely examine our daily experiences, we notice our awareness is often as follows: "I am getting this picture in my mind. I am walking. I am eating. I am thinking. I am looking at this rock, this sunset, or this automobile." Countless times a day, we acknowledge this "I" as the doer or beholder in all of our activities. This awareness of "I" is usually in relation to objects, memories, concepts, judgments, preconceptions, and more. This simple awareness of "I" is an *indirect,* as opposed to a *direct,* experience of the Self. It is indirect because it is always affected by the impressions of other materials and objects in the mind.

It is only because the mind is undisciplined, and incapable of contemplating solely on the "I" alone, that we are unable to grasp its original form. It is as if we are looking through a textured glass to see what is on the other side. What we see has been distorted by the "texture"—by the activity of the mind. If we were able to purely experience this "I" shining in the mind, then we would attain the goal of yoga. The very intention of yoga is to experience the consciousness of this "I" unconditionally, without hindrance. That itself is known as yoga.

EXPERIENCE OF ONENESS

If there is a clay pot with a light inside it, the light will illuminate only the inside of the pot. The shape of the pot will define the light's shape and scope. If we remove the pot, the light will spread out in all directions. Likewise, a spark of the Eternal Truth has entered the human system but has been covered by a veil of delusion, known as māyā. This delusion is the result of our previous births' karmas and saṃskāras. An ideal lifestyle, supported by yogic techniques, can lift this veil of delusion and allow this spark to grow into a brilliant light. This is the Soul merging with the Eternal Truth. This is the *non-dual* experience found in the highest form of Samādhi. It is why the yogic sages have defined yoga as the ultimate experience of Oneness.

UNION OF PRAKṚTI INTO PURUṢA

The whole of creation is due to two basic elements: *puruṣa* and *prakṛti*. Puruṣa refers to the Great Light, the Eternal Truth. Prakṛti is the cause of all that is manifest in this universe. Universal puruṣa, or *paramapuruṣa,* is non-dual, indivisible Oneness. Individual puruṣa is the spark of Great Light, or the individual's Soul. Universal prakṛti is the entire manifest world and universe; individual prakṛti is the body and mind.

The mind's four internal tools—manas, ahaṅkāra, mahat, and pradhāna—are part of prakṛti. When they merge into their causal state, the individual Soul will merge into the universal Soul, or paramapuruṣa, and experience an indivisible Oneness. When prakṛti merges with puruṣa, Samādhi will be experienced. For this reason, some yogis have also defined yoga as the union of prakṛti into puruṣa.

UNION OF PRĀṆA AND APĀNA

The mind and the senses are tied directly to the breath. We start breathing at birth and continue until we die. Breath is an action caused by *prāṇa* and *apāna.* They are essential for life and all external and internal activity. Prāṇa moves upward, whereas apāna drags prāṇa downward. The upward movement of prāṇa causes exhalation; the downward movement of apāna causes inhalation. Prāṇa and apāna are manifestations of a single energy split into two. If we can stop all activity—physical, as well as mental—these two energies will merge back into one. This single energy will then move upward and merge into its source. This merging mechanism of prāṇa and apāna is seen in Samādhi. Thus, yogis who experience this phenomenon have defined yoga as the union of prāṇa and apāna.

SAMATĀ

Let us try to understand one more definition of yoga. What is required to do a job properly? For a pilot to fly an airplane from one airport to another, many things must be in proper order. For example, his body should be well rested, not sleepy, tired, or hungry. His plane should be in good condition and filled with sufficient fuel. All maintenance should be performed to prevent the plane from breaking down in flight. In addition, a pilot's mind should be focused on the job at hand, free from distractions like outside business or personal problems. Furthermore, he should study the weather conditions and take off at an opportune time. He should never attempt to fly in a storm or at night, unless he has had all the proper training. If all necessary conditions are fulfilled, he will be able to safely pilot the plane.

Likewise, when we sit for meditation, all aspects of our being must cooperate. Our mind, body, and senses are all required for Realization. In fact, it is their duty to work together on this sacred journey. They are all very precious, and we need to protect them so that they will support us in our goal. If our mind has the serious intention and desire to move inward, but our senses will not relinquish their hold on the external world, our mind will only be able to move outward. Throughout the day, there are plenty of opportunities for our five senses to work and enjoy. The eyes can see many beautiful and interesting things, the ears can hear our loved ones speaking, and so on. While our senses should operate fully at appropriate times, they also ought to rest when we are sitting for meditation.

We can compare the body to a pot of water. If we want the water to be still so there are no ripples whatsoever, then we must hold the pot absolutely motionless. Likewise, meditation requires the full support of the body to remain completely still. In this sense, the mind should also support an aspirant. Its responsibilities are to maintain noble thoughts and actions, holding to the intention of Realization, and focusing resolutely on the Eternal Truth. This quest supersedes all other obligations. During meditation, the mind should forget the influences of the external world and become fully detached. It should resist the delusion that acquiring material objects will bring happiness. It should aspire to obtain this greatest possible bliss.

As we noted earlier, another term used for mahat is *buddhi*. In Saṃskṛta, *buddhi* literally means "decision," as well as "decision-making tool." In yogic theory, when the mind makes a decision, it is in the form of buddhi. *Buddhi* may also be translated as "intellect." Buddhi, or intellect, supports decision making and thus promotes action. It is greatly beneficial to our external worldly life. The intellect assists us by solving the many problems in life associated with health, education, livelihood, relationships, and responsibilities. However, it also assists us with problems associated with meditation. If the body is in pain when sitting for meditation, the intellect needs to discern some physical exercise to eliminate discomfort. If our digestion is poor, our intellect needs to ascertain the reason and determine a remedy so that the problem will not recur. In many different areas, our intellect needs to operate optimally to solve the problems that arise in our life and our practice. At its optimal capacity, the intellect leads us to one-pointed focus, which in turn leads us to Samādhi.

In the analogy of the chariot, the driver represents the intellect, the reins the mind, the five horses the senses, and the wheels and the axle represent the body. The Soul rides behind the driver and is the master of this chariot. If the driver, the horses, the wheels, and the axle all share the same intention, then the chariot will take the Soul to its destination. However, if one of the horses is unmanageable and another is lame, or a wheel is missing some spokes, then the whole system will break down. The Soul will not reach its goal. Thus, it is only when our entire system is in a state of complete cooperation that the yogic experience is possible. In yogic terms, noncooperation is *viśamatā*. Cooperation is *samatā,* and this is what is expected in the noble practitioner. Hence, yoga is defined as samatā.

THE INEXPLICABLE NATURE OF YOGA

All of the various examples mentioned above describe the same phenomenon. They simply reflect the manner in which different texts have chosen to illustrate the remarkable yogic experience. The great yogi and non-dualist philosopher Adi Shankaracharya, considered an incarnation of Śiva, viewed the yogic experience as completely unique. He explained that Samādhi is not the *waking state,* because activities are not occurring. It is not the *sleep state,* because bliss is experienced. It is not *death,* because life's activities resume after such an experience. Yet, in the deepest yogic states, one does not breathe, nor does one's blood circulate; the body is like an inert object, and no sensations are felt. However, after some time, all these activities resume one by one. After contemplating on all this, Shankaracharya concluded that the yogic experience could only be defined as something *wonderful* and *strange.*

CHAPTER FOUR

MIND AND BODY

मोक्षसाधनम्

THE NEAREST AND BEST tools to use for Realization and Liberation are our human mind and body. They are wonderful instruments. In our ancient texts the human body is referred to as an unimaginable vehicle and has been called *vimāna,* or "that which one may even use to fly"! It is also called "the wish-yielding tree," or *kalpavṛkṣa.* It is truly the grace of Nature and a microcosm of the entire universe.

Our human body is one of our most important possessions. It is the boat we use to sail the ocean of birth and death. It also comprises one of the most important set of tools we use on the yogic path, including our head, arms, and legs, as well as the brain, heart, lungs, and so on. On a deeper level, we must include our senses, intellect, and memory. It is our job to keep them all in their best possible condition.

Because it controls our entire body, the most important tool we as humans possess is our mind. If our mind is in good condition, we can *think about* how to manage any other deficiency in our body. But if our mind is in poor condition, that is not so easy. Our mind is also the most important tool on the yogic path. If we have a balanced and healthy mind, we can improve in any area where we might be deficient. We can even compensate for a total lack of competency in some area, or yogic discipline, simply through mastering another. Therefore, our first duty is to make sure our mind is in good condition. If it is not, it is our duty to discover and implement an effective and proper remedy.

Some students will look to yoga as a means to solve all their personal problems. With a proper and mature approach, this can be valid. However, just as certain physical problems require an individual to see a medical doctor, psychological problems may sometimes require an individual to see a doctor of psychology. It is our duty to use whatever corrective tools and disciplines are available to us to resolve errors that might be compromising our health. In this way, we work to create optimal health in both mind and body to benefit our yoga practice. It is ill advised to use a spiritual goal to bypass what is our duty to correct with human effort.

If Realization is the goal, one's highest priority should be to bring the mind and body into a state of perfect health and balance. "Perfect" refers to the best possible physical and mental states that support progress on the yogic path. If we lack this health and balance, it is our duty to gain it. But what constitutes perfect health and balance?

MENTAL AND PHYSICAL CONSTITUTIONS

Charcoal and diamond are both products of carbon. In the same way, everything in this universe is derived from basic constitutional elements. The ṛṣis who founded the ancient sciences of Yoga and Āyurveda identified three basic qualities, or energies, called *guṇas*. These energies are the forces underlying the *creation, maintenance,* and *destruction* of the entire universe, as well as our mind and body. They are named *sattva, rajas,* and *tamas.*

These three guṇa energies are used to describe our *mental constitution*. Each of us will contain some combination of all three guṇa energies. At the body level, these three energies are identified as *vāta*, *pitta*, and *kapha*. These are known as the three *doṣas,* and they determine our *physical constitution*. Each of us will contain some combination of all three of these, as well as the three guṇas. Our mental constitution and physical constitution influence each other. An individual's *overall* constitution is defined by all these considerations. When they are properly balanced and aligned, they define perfect health for a given individual.

THE THREE GUṆAS

Sattva energy has a tendency to move upward, toward the head. It brings calmness, quietness, and contentment. The ability to focus the mind on a single object is due to this energy. Realization of the Eternal Truth is possible through sattva.

Rajas energy moves horizontally, in an external direction, outward from the body. It carries our mind through the five senses and causes various types of voluntary and involuntary activities in our system. It is the energy for action.

Tamas energy moves downward, toward the feet. Its tendency is to cover and hide. It develops our physical body and allows us the grace of rest and sleep. While it causes ignorance, it can also shield us from negative and traumatic experiences. The ignorance that arises from tamas energy develops the attachment that holds us to this birth and death cycle.

Every single thing in the universe possesses all three of these energies. However, the proportion will vary from object to object and from individual to individual. One may be sattva dominant, or *sattvic*. Another may be rajas dominant, or *rajasic*. A third may be tamas dominant, or *tamasic*. Some individuals will be dual natured; for example, they may be primarily sattvic, but partially rajasic. In this way, fourteen different combinations are derived.

The human body contains a number of *astral channels* called *nāḍīs*. These nāḍīs allow movement of the three guṇa energies. Most nāḍīs channel these guṇa energies in external directions, either horizontally or downward. However, one, located along our spine, permits an internal upward movement toward the higher spheres. As sattva moves in this upward direction, our mind moves inward. (Likewise, as our mind moves inward, sattva moves upward.) This is why the upright position of our spine is absolutely essential for Realization. Our vertical backbone is uniquely oriented from that of other living beings. While animals and birds can move their minds only in the outward direction, human beings can move their minds in either direction. This is possible only due to the grace of Nature in endowing our body with a vertical spine.

THREE KINGS TO RULE IN HARMONY

When the three guṇa energies work together in harmony, they beget many noble qualities, such as sympathy, love, compassion, patience, and wit, all of which are seen in ideal human beings. However, human beings possess a unique predilection toward sattva energy, while other animals are rajas dominant and vegetation is tamas dominant.

As per yogic philosophy, noble qualities or attributes are also known as guṇas because they help us reach the final goal. For instance, in a healthy human being, the energy of sattva will develop the qualities of compassion and mercy. A sattvic mind can easily understand the pain of others and, to almost any extent, it can find remedies for that pain. Because compassion is so closely associated with sattva, compassion itself is labeled as a guṇa. Rajasic energy sparks enthusiasm and an adventurous nature in a healthy mind. Because enthusiasm and a spirit of adventure are noble qualities, they, too, are termed guṇas. Likewise, tamasic energy helps us forget traumatic incidents that may otherwise be unbearable to hold in our minds. This kind of beneficial forgetfulness may be labeled as a guṇa. All human beings are capable of developing these attributes, or guṇas. They account for that which is noble and enlightened in human beings. To reach the final target, we need these attributes. My Eternal Teacher, Śrī Raṅga, explained it in this way: "This human kingdom is well managed by these three kings. When they rule in harmony, and in a full understanding with one another, there will be total health in our system."

THE GATEWAY WITHIN

Our body is a gateway to a wonderful world within. Our body is divine. All the organs in this complicated and elaborate system are divine. All of its parts, each playing an important role in providing us with proper health, are divine. Even the smallest hair plays a role in our health and well-being. Most yogic disciplines focus directly and indirectly on maintaining the perfect health of mind and body so that we can move inward to the divine spheres. Because this mind and body are so very, very precious, we are wise to avoid burdening them excessively. If we torture this system, it will lose its capacity for Realization and Liberation. We need to direct our full energy and attention toward maintaining our mind and body in the absolute best possible condition. To achieve optimum health, there are guidelines to follow for even the simplest of activities, such as washing our body and handling various objects and materials. If this mind and body are in perfect condition, Liberation will be found naturally. We need not struggle.

BENEFITS OF LESS STRAIN

An important guiding principle of yoga encourages us to live in this world without straining our system. Our first duty as a human being upon awakening is to sit for a little while and assess our mind and body. It is helpful to conduct a mental inventory of our body to compare its state of health to that of the day before. Also, we can try to take an objective look at our mind. Are we upset about anything, or is our mind in a calm and quiet condition? If we are stressed or unwell in any way, it is our responsibility to rectify this. This is an essential point. If we do not strain our system, our body will inevitably come to a balanced condition and stay that way.

If we observe other animals living in their natural habitat, we will see that they live by this principle. For the most part, they proceed through life without undue struggle. Of course, they may struggle at times to find food, but this mostly occurs when their habitat is disturbed. Generally, they pass their time with ease. They may wander here and there in search of food. They may drink water at a pond or a stream. They may lie down and rest in the shade of a tree. Their way of life has an even, uncomplicated quality about it. This is also the best way for us to live—simply and easily, like an animal in its natural environment. There is a Saṃskṛta phrase for this sort of way of life: *anāyāsena jīvanam,* meaning the human life without strain.

Although few can live by simply gathering food in the forest, we can still choose to live a simple life. It is enough to have some meaningful work that brings in adequate money to provide food and shelter. If we constantly crave more and more material possessions, a simple job will not be sufficient. But if we eliminate that craving and focus on what is most important, we can likely find a vocation that will supply our needs. As a result, we will have plenty of spare time to attend to yogic disciplines and practices. If we spend these hours preparing and consuming precious food, engaging in proper and light exercise, and practicing various other yogic disciplines—all with the intent of achieving Realization and Liberation—we are attending to what is most precious in life, and our most fundamental duty. However, if we spend our free time watching television or engaged in other trivial pursuits, we are not using our time properly. These things end up being forms of escapism. Much of this is totally meaningless. In the end, we will come to realize that they have offered us little in return for our time and energy.

YOGIC SIGHT

When we explore any aspect of yoga, we must maintain sight of its ultimate purposes, which are Samādhi and Realization. All of the yogic and related Indian sciences owe their existence to the calm and quiet mind experienced through Samādhi and Realization. For example, there are sixty-four Indian sciences, and each has evolved through yogic sight, serving humankind in its own way. These disciplines include dance, music, mathematics, astrology, Āyurveda, and so on. Each will attract a particular individual based on her constitution. However, the single goal of all sixty-four sciences is Samādhi and Realization. The correct study of any one of these sciences will remind us of their ultimate purpose. Using the proper technique, we can discover many hidden secrets in the universe. If we know these secrets, we can use worldly materials for their correct and intended purpose. Thus, we will find it easy to solve many problems.

The ability to look deeply into objects, materials, and substances found throughout the universe aids us in maintaining our own health, as well as the health of those around us. When the yogic experience eliminates the mind's preconditioning, we gain the ability to contemplate deeply on any aspect of the universe. This is what is meant by *yogic sight.* If one chooses, and Nature permits, one's mind can penetrate into any object or material and fully grasp the underlying truth and essence of that object or material.

In this way, one can visualize anything through yogic sight and, in most cases, Nature will allow someone with an unconditioned mind to discover her secrets. However, sometimes, for the welfare of all humankind, Nature chooses to cover even the mind of the Realized. A yogi may sit and meditate on some subject and realize in the process of the meditation, "No, this cannot be understood. Nature's intention is to keep this subject hidden."

The yogic experience will also benefit our memory. When the yogic experience brings calmness and quietness, we easily record in our mind whatever we see and understand. We develop a wonderful memory and capacity to recollect things at any time.

Long ago when many of the early texts were being shared, instead of using many books, it was common practice for scholars to memorize a text in its entirety. In this way, individuals memorized the entire Vedas—ancient eternal teachings conveying the nature of the universe, Soul, and Eternal Truth. Even today our mind has this capacity, but most of us do not exercise it. Instead, we rely on writing, books, and smartphones. In fact, the sages of today say that it is because of our reliance on all these devices that our memory has faded.

In fact, the stories within the *Mahābhārata* describe many advanced yogis or yoga practitioners. People living at that time had calm and quiet minds, as well as capacities that, by today's standards, would seem magical and fantastic. There are accounts of people being able to see great distances, recite potent *mantras,* and even fly great distances. Today, there are people who still possess such amazing powers. Those who have seen such yogis and sages living today can give credence to the ancient stories. Even if we do not accept such stories, we can still benefit from their underlying messages.

The power of a yogi's intellect and memory are directly related to the calmness and quietness of his mind. Of course, not all yogis have the same innate capacity. Some will have more and some less based on their constitution. However, when a practitioner is regularly experiencing yogic conditions, his memory and intellect will increase to the maximum extent allowed by his constitution.

EFFECTS ON OUR HEALTH

Yogic practices deeply affect our state of health in mind and body. Most psychological and physical disorders are of two categories. One is rooted in incorrect behavior in this birth. The other is caused by an error in a previous birth. If treated early enough, most disorders caused by the errors in this birth will be solved by proper medicine. Their sources are not deeply rooted when compared with more serious disorders that arise from karma and deeply ingrained saṃskāras from previous births.

We may have a chronic health problem and try many medicines to cure it, but due to ongoing disturbances in our mind, nothing provides the cure. For example, hyperacidity is a problem where the stomach produces more gastric secretions than necessary. One who suffers from this will feel a burning sensation and the secretions may cause ulcers. Through a calm and quiet mind, a yoga practitioner brings balance to his digestive system. He will naturally correct his eating habits, and his digestive system will then activate at the right time every day. The effects of yogic conditions may fully correct this disease, and the practitioner will no longer suffer.

The yogic experience can also lessen the effects of deeply rooted disorders caused by wrong actions in previous births. There are two aspects of these disorders that may affect a person's mind or body. One is the actual karma-induced problem; the other is a person's psychological reaction to that problem. This reaction stems from the person's ignorance and aversion as to why he has experienced such a disorder in this lifetime. This psychological reaction can greatly increase a person's suffering—even doubling the effects of a karma-induced problem. The experience of the Eternal Truth eliminates all of these psychological disturbances. The remaining karmic-induced problems may then become bearable. We can then accept that we made some error in a past life for which we must simply bear the repercussions.

For example, eczema is a disorder that causes inflammation of the skin. It causes a disturbing itching sensation that constantly drags the sufferer's attention to it. One must often apply medicine to relieve the itching. In some cases, this disease also brings psychological problems. One who suffers from this disease often feels shame about his appearance and constantly worries about it. His worrying, in effect, doubles the problem, creating much more misery. This misery is created by his mind, not by the disease. According to Āyurvedic medicine, eczema is a problem that can be solved, though it may require many years of effort. With that same effort, one might achieve Self-Realization, and thereby solve all his problems! Therefore, yogis consider that it is better to simply apply some creams and medicine to relieve the minor symptoms and spend one's primary effort on attaining Self-Realization.

A basic principle of the universe is that there are remedies for all problems, but often our minds are not capable of thinking properly in the direction where we will find the remedy. Sometimes we work too much. Sometimes we do not eat properly. Sometimes we have relationship problems. All these things cause our minds and bodies to suffer. The biggest problem, the root problem, however, is that we are not happy. We have not satisfied our deep craving for internal peace, happiness, and bliss. This is all because we have not experienced the Eternal Truth. For this, one should balance and purify the mind and body by living an ideal way of life.

THE NATURAL CALL FOR QUIETNESS

Nature provides us with signs to experience the yogic state of Samādhi, but we have lost our ability to recognize them. We are so unaccustomed to this particular calm and quiet bliss that, even if we do feel it, we usually fail to stop and let it affect us. However, if we continue to ignore the messages that are coming our way, we may even lose our capacity to receive them.

For instance, we naturally feel hunger at a particular time each day. If we ignore our appetite by busying ourselves with other activities, our body will gradually adjust and we will no longer feel hunger at that time. If we continue this pattern long enough, then even when we are not occupied, we will not be hungry. By disrupting the body's cycle, we end up depriving it of the nourishment it naturally craves.

The joy of Samādhi has different characteristics than joy from external sources. It brings a unique quality of quietness and lightness. Happiness that originates from the outside is not only limited in quantity but also develops further cravings and thus causes imbalance in our system.

A natural call to quiet the mind comes regularly around sunrise, sunset, and, to a lesser extent, at noontime and midnight. If we examine nature at dawn and dusk, we can observe certain phenomena. For instance, the wind tends to die down and leaves of trees frequently fall silent. Many animals will even stop their activities. At these times, if we keenly observe our mind, we will begin to notice fewer thoughts.

Although we have fewer thoughts at these hours, they are not eliminated. They continue to occur because we have not cultivated the practice of keeping our mind quiet.

Nonetheless, the appearance of these signs at regular times each day is in harmony with the natural cycles of our own body and mind. This observation supports the view that the yogic state is a natural state for us. If we systematically and intentionally allow our mind to abide in stillness every day, morning and evening, then our mind will naturally become relaxed. Soon we will discover the presence of a kind of spontaneous joy emerging. When we become conscious of these dynamics and allow them to influence our system, it will help us on our yogic path and eventually guide us toward the experience of Samādhi.

A VEHICLE FOR FLIGHT

The ancient sages possessed wonderful and fantastic powers of both mind and body. In the Indian epic, the Rāmāyaṇa, there is an episode in which Rāma flies from Sri Lanka to Ayodhya, an ancient city in India. The story explains what he saw as he flew, describing the various mountains, valleys, rivers, as well as both green and arid lands. The sages claim that human beings had actually developed the capacity to fly. According to the ancient texts, they used an entirely different device from the modern airplane, which they called *vimāna,* which translates roughly as "vehicle for flight." Unlike the airplane, however, this mechanism was powered by the human mind!

This is why the sages applied this word *vimāna* to the human mind and body. With the support of our body, we can use our mind as a vehicle for the yogic journey. As something akin to an airplane, our mind and body allow us to fly to inner worlds and higher spheres. This possibility is unique to human beings. If we recognize our mind and body to be aids on the path to Realization, we will love them accordingly. We will not act in a destructive manner toward them. We will avoid generating the saṃskāra that causes rebirth. If we love this mind and body, our vehicle, we will keep it clean. If it needs any small repair, we will attend to it immediately. At the same time, it is only a borrowed vehicle, so we will use it simply as a tool. Later, when we reach our destination, we will leave it behind and move on. We will not be further concerned about or attached to it. To have yogic experiences, it is imperative that we forget this body completely. That is possible only if we love it meaningfully.

CHAPTER FIVE

THE HUMAN PREDICAMENT

मनुजगतिः

OUR MIND has unlimited potential. But if we truly possess such great potential, why do we not always see this universe, and our own role in it, clearly? Our mind is hindered to the extent that we are unable to view the universe without the influence of our prior conditioning. Lacking an unconditioned perspective, we cannot correctly assess the ultimate purpose of our mind and body. Nor do we often correctly assess the proper use of the material world. This limited vision is found in nearly all human beings and misleads many human endeavors and journeys, including the most sophisticated sciences.

There is a divine energy at work supporting this entire universe. Through the ages, great sages have used their yogic sight to better understand the mysterious workings of this energy. Through close observation, they have come to understand this as māyā, divine energy that exists to both cover and shield the Eternal Truth. This energy leads to the basic workings of karma and saṃskāra. Together, these three principles are part of the divine law that shapes our lives. They work together to determine our fate and are themselves determined by our human effort. It is through the yogic experience that we gain knowledge and awareness of how these principles operate in our lives. With this insight, we can take the appropriate measures to lessen their negative impact and free ourselves from the vicious cycles that may otherwise ensue. Thus, we free ourselves from the conditioning that prevents us from accurately and objectively viewing this universe. When we do so, we gradually free ourselves from our human predicament and come to experience the full potential of our body and mind.

MĀYĀ

Everything in this universe can either support or hinder us in experiencing the non-dual Oneness of the Eternal Truth. Māyā is the screen that exists between "reality" and Realization. It is a divine energy that exists to both cover and shield the Eternal Truth. As such, it both supports and hinders us in achieving Realization. Yoga explains that māyā itself is prakṛti—the divine energy that supports the unfolding of all that is manifest in the universe. It provides us with all the wonderful forms that comprise the physical world, but we must remember that this is not in itself the ultimate Truth.

KARMA

To some degree we act as we choose in life. This freedom often causes us difficulty. Our actions can bring either balance or unwanted consequences. When we lose our balance, Nature attempts to correct our mistakes, letting us experience the pain, misery, or good that result from these actions. This is the basic principle of karma. In Saṃskṛta, *karma* primarily means "action." It is also referred to as *adṛṣṭa*—an unseen cause that brings pleasure and pain as the consequence of our good and bad deeds. The reason we do not always fully understand the link between our actions and their resultant misery or joy is māyā's influence.

SAṂSKĀRA

Saṃskāra refers to deeply ingrained patterns of thought or behavior. These patterns can be like ruts in a poor road that prevent us from altering our course, or they can fully support us, like a smooth freeway that helps us travel quickly to our destination. Like karma, saṃskāra can be either positive or negative. Negative saṃskāras create bondage through wrong deeds. Positive saṃskāras support our health and well-being. They lead us to understand the Truth and lead us in the direction of the Realization of the Self.

THE INTERACTION OF MĀYĀ AND KARMA

As free agents, we are fully responsible for our actions. Therefore, we must eventually reap their full benefit or pay their full cost. It is the role of māyā to assist us in this transaction. At appropriate times, māyā covers the mind so that we cannot properly understand the true nature of reality. In doing so, it allows us to act in certain ways so karma can unfold and bring its results.

For example, if we perform some misdeed, we must eventually suffer a corrective consequence of that action. If we do not immediately experience some pain or corrective measure, we will be led to do so at a later time, or even later in life. We will eventually act in some way that leads us to suffer for our misdeed. If we saw this coming, we would likely try to avoid the personal pain that was our due. However, through māyā, a screen of delusion will obscure our understanding in that moment. We will then unknowingly act in such a way that allows the corrective karma to unfold.

Māyā can also act as a shield to protect us at times from making errors. It does this by also limiting our awareness, thereby reducing the chance that we will commit even worse mistakes. For example, a person might be walking down a street toward a place where he could end up engaging in some negative behavior. Māyā can protect that person by causing him to walk elsewhere, thus avoiding that particular situation. In this way, the divine energy of māyā guides us through life so that we avoid creating further negative karma and our actions may support us in positive ways. Moreover, if one has a strong intention for Liberation, māyā has the capacity to cover the external world, thus limiting its attractive nature and apparent allure.

THE INTERACTION OF MĀYĀ AND SAṂSKĀRA

Māyā is also what leads us to develop certain tendencies and biases. The mind's tendency toward bias is caused by attachments and aversions that obscure objective observation. Gradually, a filter arises so that nothing is seen as it is. For example, our eyes tell us that water is colorless, milk is white, and crows are black. However, if we put a red filter in front of our eyes, the color of everything changes. If we consistently keep that filter in place, we become accustomed to it; we think that reality is what we perceive through the filter. Later, when we remove the filter, we feel something is wrong with our eyes. If we hold a particular thought or attitude long enough, we end up believing it. We lose the ability to distinguish the truth. This is also the work of māyā, creator of the mind's conditioning.

A young girl might hear that yogurt is made from a type of bacteria and develop a strong aversion to it. She may think that it is spoiled and unfit to eat. Even if her parents and older brothers and sisters show her that it is good to eat, she will not eat it. She may even read about the health benefits of yogurt, and still she cannot enjoy it. It is her prior conditioning that prevents her from enjoying it.

A boy may observe his father behaving in a miserly way. Perhaps the father is always grasping for money, bargaining harshly with everybody, and never spending anything unless he is forced to do so. The boy may soon imitate his father and develop the same behavior. Later in life, when he encounters a charitable person, he will not appreciate that person's generosity. Even if the benefits of sharing and generosity are vividly demonstrated to him, he will not understand. This, too, is because of prior conditioning.

We are all familiar with childhood conditioning, but that is not the strongest force. The conditioning we bring from our past lives is far stronger. This is the conditioning of saṃskāra. It is like a seed carried in our mind from previous births. This seed then produces direct, or indirect, repercussions out of the actions of our previous births. These repercussions lead us to act in ways that develop even more karma and deepen the saṃskāra.

Most often, our inappropriate actions are a direct result of the ignorance that results from māyā's screen of delusion. These actions cause our problems not only in this life, but also from one birth to the next. In past lives, we may have misused a certain material through a lack of understanding. Nature demands that we reap the results of this misuse. The errors from our previous births will lead māyā to create delusion in this one. The delusion that thus results will cause us to suffer the consequences of those previous errors. Furthermore, our delusions steer us toward multiple misguided actions, which perpetuate a cyclical pattern. Our conditioning develops out of this vicious cycle. This is another way māyā creates a screen of delusion and influence. In doing that, māyā plays a central role in predetermining our next births. This is a very difficult cycle to escape, though sincere human effort and practice has the power to change its course.

THE UNCONDITIONED MIND

An unconditioned mind is capable of seeing things as they are, objectively and with a fresh eye in each moment. Each observation about oneself, or the world, can be made anew without preconceptions. For example, if a person clearly understands the proper use for a particular object, it will not only benefit her in this life, but also provide a positive impression in her next birth. Consequently, her life will be more balanced and happy because of that saṃskāra.

Some level of karma and saṃskāra grips the mind of every human being. There are those who are plagued with an intense degree of conditioning, while others are born with less. Very few, like the incarnations Rāma and Kṛṣṇa, have none whatsoever. For the most part, even those who are Realized must live out their karma and saṃskāra from previous births. Due to their total awareness and deep insight into the nature of the universe, however, they no longer become attached to their actions. Therefore, a Realized person's actions will not acquire new karmas or saṃskāras. This is because karma relies on our attachment to continue the cycle from birth to birth. Attachment is like water for the seed of a previous karma to grow. Without attachment, all karma loses its sustenance. Once a Realized person leaves their body, they will not be reborn. They will be Liberated.

However, for most human beings, karma and saṃskāra shape the next birth, so that they will receive the results of their actions and fulfill their desires. In one way, our mind is unimaginably powerful. Our wants and wishes must come to fruition. There is a cliché that warns, "Be careful what you wish for—you just might get it." Yogic philosophy claims, "Mind is the wish-yielding tree," so, therefore, "Be mindful about your desires, for they will certainly manifest in this birth or the next."

KARMA AND ITS RESULTS

We might ask, *"Why don't our current actions always give their results in this life?"* It must be understood that every action yields its own unique results. Right now, in this life, both karma and saṃskāras are operating from our previous births. If the results of our present actions are not in conflict with these two principles, we will see the results in this incarnation.

For example, karma from a previous birth may be forcing us to act in a way that leads us to suffer a psychological or physical disorder. If we perform some action unrelated to this karma, and if the result of that action can coexist with this disorder, we can experience both karmas in this birth simultaneously. However, if these karmas somehow conflict with one another, we may not see the full consequences in this lifetime; one karma may be postponed for another opportunity to unfold in a later birth—unless we avoid them completely by achieving Realization in this birth.

For instance, we may be performing actions that should bring us prosperity. We are using money wisely, including being generous in appropriate ways. However, the results of our past life may still be running their course and demand that we experience poverty. It is the time for that particular karma to run its course. It may even need an entire lifetime or longer to be cleared. This is why right actions in this birth must often wait for a later birth to experience their full results.

However, a very powerful good or bad deed will provide its result in this life itself. An example might be if a person takes great risk to save others in a fire or storm. Surely, this person will be honored and receive some karmic results in this lifetime. Even greater still are the karmic results when a person saves another who himself is Realized. That is a very powerful deed. Its karmic results will certainly appear in this very life.

Yoga says that there are answers to every problem. If we know those solutions and work hard, we can make progress. Sometimes, if we are determined enough, we will find ways to overcome a very persistent disorder. However, sometimes our determination is not enough. If an illness has karmic roots, we can try to apply all known remedies but receive little or no benefit. Sometimes the remedy may be extremely complicated and difficult, while the disorder is relatively minor. Then the cure may be worse than the disease. In such cases, it is better to accept the disorder. Do what can be done easily and make peace with it. Though we are poor, if we are healthy, have enough to eat, a good roof over our head, and are able to practice yoga, we should accept our fate and not struggle too hard against it.

GRACE OF THE ETERNAL TRUTH

I was born in a small village where my father was a Saṃskṛta scholar and known speaker. He was also part of a family lineage that practiced the science of Vedic astrology for many generations. This knowledge was considered a hereditary gift, and it was our family's duty to provide this service to all. For our primary livelihood, however, we depended on farming. We raised cows and grew rice, bananas, areca, and other small crops.

While in high school, I was a good speaker and had a knack for science. All my teachers encouraged me to go on to study science. However, my father was totally against this. He wanted me to study Saṃskṛta and astrology. This was the tradition, and he was firm in his thinking.

My father was a very strict man, and I never disobeyed him. As a result, I was forced to study Saṃskṛta and attend a traditional school, or *pāṭhaśālā,* at Shringeri, a place famous for its association with the great non-dual philosopher Adi Shankaracharya. Here I studied secondary Saṃskṛta lessons with a teacher named Ganesha Shastry. He was a very good Saṃskṛta scholar and very knowledgeable in Āyurveda. In addition, he was a poet and an advanced spiritual practitioner. I honored him as my heartfelt teacher.

After I had studied Saṃskṛta for two years, my father's plan was for me to study astrology in Udupi, a town not far from my birthplace and famous for astrology. With pride, my father made arrangements for my studies. All this time, I did not have the desire or the heart to study astrology. However, I decided to follow my father's wishes and go to Udupi.

I happened to have a close friend who was going to Mysore to continue his studies. He and I decided we would depart on the same date to travel our separate ways. When that day arrived, we both went to salute our teacher and get his final blessing. We offered him flowers, some fruits, and a small donation, or *gurudakṣiṇā*. My teacher knew I was going to study astrology. He also knew my father. But when I raised my head, having saluted him, he unexpectedly said, "Shankaranarayana, whatever your father may say, I feel you should go to Mysore! As your teacher, this is my intuition. I don't know why I feel this way, but I am sure your prosperity will be in Mysore and not Udupi. Your father will likely get very upset, but you must find a way to convince him of this decision."

I found myself completely stunned. I had been raised with the belief that one should honor and obey both father and teacher. When their words contradict each other, however, tradition also says one should follow the teacher. At that moment, I decided to go against my father's wish. When my friend and I got to the bus station, we both boarded the bus to Mysore.

At the time, it was not clear to me why or how I made that decision on that day. Later, I understood what a significant turning point this was in my life. I am now certain that the grace of the Eternal Truth convinced my teacher to direct me on that fateful day. As a result of that decision, I was led to the very person who would become my Eternal Teacher and guide for the rest of my life—the great yogi Śrī Raṅga. Whenever I think of this, my heart melts with enormous gratitude for the honorable Śrī Ganesha Shastry, who worked as a channel for the Divine.

FATE AND HUMAN EFFORT

Yogic philosophy never asserts that everything is fixed by fate. We are not puppets in the drama of life. Moreover, the word *fate* is commonly used to describe that which is inevitable, predetermined, and completely out of our control. According to yoga philosophy, this is not an entirely accurate definition. In fact, fate arises from the actions of our previous births. Like māyā, fate allows for the unfolding of karma in our lives. Fate follows the divine law of cause and effect. In this way, it is known as *daiva,* the supporting principle of this entire universe. Because it lies hidden in the actions of our past lives, the *cause* of our fate is impossible for most people to understand. Hence, it feels mysteriously predetermined and "out of our control."

What we do control is our human effort. We know that whatever action we take, we will experience the results eventually—either in this life or in the next. Human effort will always yield its results. The question we must ask is How might we direct our human effort in ways that do not create negative karma and saṃskāra?

Quite often, people mistakenly conclude that their efforts are a failure. This is because they do not properly assess the karma that is currently operating in their lives. If they have made a prodigious effort with no visible results, they might complain, "Oh, what a waste of time this has been. After all that energy, there is nothing to show for it."

It is very difficult to understand fully and accurately the complex dynamics of karma currently at work in our lives. Even though we may not be able to enjoy the benefits immediately, it is our duty to perform right actions. We need to be very patient about experiencing the results. This mechanism of daiva, or fate, works in its own time. This should not discourage us from doing our duty.

If we cannot assess which karma is currently operating, or what the outcome of our actions will be, then we certainly cannot predict when or how our efforts will unfold. This is one of many reasons it is far better not to expect results from our actions. If we are not attached to the results of our actions, then we need not worry about our current karma. We should simply try to do our duty, and let that be enough. If we learn to act without expectation, we will not be disappointed. What is more, we will feel more balanced in our lives. We will reap the results at some future time.

Fate and human effort are like two wheels of a chariot. We should maintain each in a well-balanced manner. Trusting in human effort alone develops egotism; surrendering to fate alone prevents one from performing his duty. A wise person will account for both equally.

CAN KARMA BE NULLIFIED?

There will be contradictory actions in every person's life. A man may abuse and hurt one person and help another at some other time. If someone does something harmful in her life and later performs some act of kindness, will these two actions nullify each other? Will they both provide karma for the future? Or will there be some old karma partially remaining? What will be the net karmic result?

This depends in large part on the *intentions* that lie behind our actions. Normally, because we do not intend for one action to negate another, we will experience the results of both deeds separately. However, if nullification is our intention, then it will be so, providing the opposing actions are equal in measure. A man may have stolen some items as a youth. Later, he may seriously repent for his deeds. He may find the victim of his theft and ask for forgiveness and offer compensation. If it is impossible to find the victim, he may help others in need with money or food, with an intention to rectify his errors.

Perhaps as a teenager, a person was cruel to animals. Later in life, an appropriate counterbalance would be to regularly offer food to hungry animals. If this action is performed with an intention to offer mercy for such violence, it will nullify the negative karma. Good deeds may be done specifically to make amends for previous harmful deeds. If the intention is to cancel out the effects of those actions, and if the corrective action is performed in adequate measure, it will erase the effects of the previous transgressions. But such corrective action should be very meaningful; otherwise, both results will be carried to the next birth. Practices including penance, fasting, and chanting are all considered powerful corrective actions that can nullify the effects of negative karma.

Disorders call for treatment. If we treat a disorder, it may or may not respond. If it does respond, some aspect of the disorder may be effectively treated, while another aspect continues to disturb us. This is because there is a lack of appropriate intention to cancel out the actions that originally caused the disorder. In such cases, the karma will not be canceled and will continue to deliver its results. In contrast, if our intention is to cancel the results of a previous misguided deed, and we take meaningful action, the correction will be more effective. As we have explained, however, māyā will often shield us from understanding which previous actions have caused our current disorders. With this lack of clear understanding, we may not be able to move ahead with the right intention. This will be common until we have developed insight into our true Self. Until then, we should seek the guidance of a knowledgeable person.

These are all simply corrective measures. However, in order to shield ourselves from acquiring more negative karma in our life, we should adopt a meaningful approach to all our daily actions. Simply put, Do your duty. Perform whatever right actions life requires, then surrender these actions and their results to the Divine. In other words, whatever the results may be, enjoy them, or at the very least, simply accept them.

Right actions will work collectively to nullify this life's karma that may be dragging you down. They bring harmony to the system. This harmony itself will support Liberation. This is considered the optimal approach to our endeavors. Still, we may be left with many questions. How do we achieve such results? What is the best route for us to transcend our human predicament? What can we do to experience Samādhi and be delivered from the cycle of birth and death?

LIFE'S MOST IMPORTANT DUTIES

None of us come into this life entirely on our own. We are the offspring of our mother and father, and they the offspring of their parents. In addition, we all have many connections to other people, places, and aspects of the material world. Wherever we are linked, we are also hooked in a certain way. Our lives are like a spider's web. If one thread is pulled, the whole web will change shape. Thus, we are not totally independent; rather, we share responsibility for others and the world around us. This is what underlies the concept of duty.

It is our duty and responsibility to think of the welfare of those related to us. First come mother and father, then grandfather and grandmother, and then other blood relations. Next, our duty is to those with whom we share a deep heart connection. If we marry, a commitment and heart connection should be established with our spouse. If a couple has a child, they become even more powerfully linked through that child. One may also be closely linked with friends, coworkers, employees, well-wishers, neighbors, and so on. For a variety of reasons, we may love these people, and they, too, show love and affection toward us. We may even feel a particular appreciation for the village or town where we were born, or a place where we have lived a very long time. There is an implicit recognition that these places have served us, so we feel indebtedness toward them. Many people feel a strong link and connectedness to nature and what the natural world provides in terms of beauty and resources for our daily sustenance. If we have developed a connection to the divine, we may feel a love in our heart for that particular grace or deity. We must acknowledge and attend to all these many relationships and connections if our goal is to live a noble and ideal life. This is our duty.

Duty means "that which must be done"—otherwise, it will have a negative impact on our lives in the form of karma. It is like a contractual commitment one cannot escape. When we borrow money, we make a commitment to pay it back at some point. Likewise, each person born owes a kind of debt, or obligation, to Nature for all that life affords us. This is known as *ṛṇa.* There are three important ruṇas we must understand: *deva ṛṇa, pitṛ ṛṇa,* and *ṛṣi ṛṇa.*

DEVA ṚṆA

Deva ṛṇa is the obligation we have to certain energies working throughout our system. These energies operate through many subtle branches and are affected by our actions. Yogis call these energies *deities.* One pleases and honors these energies, or deities, by acknowledging the ways in which they support our existence and by showing them gratitude. This is what is meant by true worship. When we do this, we perform *yajña*, acts of worship and sacrifice. This may be done through penance, fasting, chanting, prāṇāyāma, and so on. Performing yajña repays the debt we owe these divine energies for the many benefits they provide us in our daily lives. Such actions facilitate these energies to work favorably in our system and eliminate our deva ṛṇa.

PITṚ ṚṆA

We are the offspring of our father and mother, and they of their parents. Along with our brothers and sisters, we share innumerable links with our parents. The most obvious is our physical body, which even shares the same DNA. Pitṛ ṛṇa is the debt we owe to our parents for this life, their love, and their care. We fulfill this obligation by serving and honoring them during their lifetime, and even after their death. There are many ways we can honor our parents. One is by showing them gratitude. However, the greatest way we honor our parents is by having noble children ourselves. Children are the new sprouts of our family tree. They come through the grace of pitṛ energy. Having children is one of the most powerful ways to eliminate pitṛ ṛṇa. A person who chooses not to have children, or cannot conceive children, may eliminate pitṛ ṛṇa by turning their focus entirely on achieving Realization.

ṚṢI ṚṆA

As human beings, we have the capacity to understand who we truly are, life's purpose, and the universe. We learn the answers to these questions according to our constitution and individual capacity. However, this education is not likely to come through our studies in school or college. We are more likely to gain this wisdom through hearing the words of knowledgeable teachers. If we are so fortunate, it becomes our duty to focus on this knowledge, setting a target of Realization. The debt we owe for all that guides us on our path toward Realization is ṛṣi ṛṇa. We honor this obligation by honoring the teachings, focusing on the Soul, and fully embracing our yogic path. In short, this is *brahmacarya*—moving toward Realization—a concept we will explain in part two of this book when discussing the *yamas*.

These three ṛṇa, and their far-reaching implications, underlie the basic understanding of duty. No one can escape these obligations. It is a contract with Nature. Duty is a commitment we take at our birth. It is a hook that tethers us in this life. Unless we perform these actions with a proper understanding, we cannot be released from these contracts. Until we are released, Liberation is not possible. Only a true renunciate will not be bound by such obligations. If an ordinary person tries to escape from them, they will be caught one way or another.

Eliminating these ṛṇa will lead to internal and external growth. It will even facilitate healthy enjoyment of the material world and lead individuals to prosperity to the degree that their karma and human effort permit. In this way, even their material prosperity will support Realization.

DUTY AND SPIRITUAL LIFE

Some people ignore their day-to-day responsibilities in life. They believe they need not attend to various mundane duties because they are living a "spiritual life" and therefore must remain detached. They might avoid looking for meaningful work or taking care of their families. Often, they will burden others with their needs. Some may live in an āśrama or join other organizations to avoid a certain level of accountability. Even then, they may unknowingly be caught by many attachments. If they are not practicing true detachment, they are spiritually bypassing their true responsibilities and their ṛṇa. These responsibilities are an important part of spiritual life. Duty is like a tollgate collecting a fee for all the many benefits we have received in our life. If it is not paid, we will not only be held accountable at some point, but we will accumulate additional karma as a corrective measure. This, in itself, may lead to additional suffering and struggle.

Therefore, it is better that we recognize where our true responsibilities lie and be honest about our attachment tendencies. We should never feel that it is a waste of time and energy to fulfill these obligations. The more we take them to heart and attend to them, the more they will help us on our path toward Realization. With proper understanding, we will more easily and quickly realize the Eternal Truth. All aspirants should know and understand this particular relationship to the Divine so that it becomes meaningful to their lives and yoga practice.

DUTY AND ATTACHMENT

How can we attend to all of these duties with whole-heartedness and yet maintain little or no attachment? Are not these links and connections forms of attachment themselves?

Duty is a commitment without attachment. For instance, all day long a bank teller may be involved with receiving and handing out money. This is his duty. He will not suddenly get sad if someone withdraws a large sum of money, nor will he be happy if someone makes a huge deposit. Even though he performs these transactions with his full commitment and involvement, he does not get attached to them. If approached like this, duty will not bind us in any way.

Imbalance in one form or another is the telltale sign of an incorrect attachment. For instance, a woman having great wealth may believe her survival is threatened if her money is lost or stolen. This simply reveals her over-attachment to money. As a result, she may behave in ways that are injurious to herself and those around her. However, money is not the same thing as happiness; it is very possible to enjoy life fully without money. Moreover, many people with a lot of money have no enjoyment at all in their lives. Equating money with happiness is erroneous, caused by attachment, and produces destructive behavior.

OPEN-HEARTED APPROACH

There are right and wrong ways to approach all our duties in life. If one feels resentment or reluctance while performing his duty, it is considered incomplete and some karma will linger. For instance, if we have a child, it is not only our duty to feed and clothe her properly, but it is also our duty to love her and show her our affection. A child's growth and health are due to many factors that help develop necessary emotional balance. All duty should be done with this kind of full and open heart. It is best done with love, affection, sincere interest, honor, and humility. Then our sincere effort will not only serve others, it will also greatly serve our own path toward Liberation.

LOVE AND ATTACHMENT

Two words in Saṃskṛta, *prīti* and *prema,* denote a particular kind of love found in life. Nearly synonymous, they refer to the kind of heart opening that links us with the internal world, bringing great joy and happiness in the process. When we are walking in a garden, we might see a beautiful flower and feel a flow of appreciation and love for it. This flower is there for us by the grace of Nature. When we love that flower in a pure way, we are honoring the grace of Nature. As this grace begins to flow from inside of us, we feel a natural type of joy. Loving something in this sense is not attachment. Rather, when we correctly view the object of our love, it becomes a form of detachment; we see it as emanating from the Divine, not as belonging to us. We come to understand that all things we love are manifestations of the grace of Nature.

We may experience great love for our spouse, children, teacher, friends, and relations, even our house and work, yet remain detached. In fact, real love is an appreciation of something or someone without attachment. *Prīti* and *prema* refer to love where there is no expectation love where there is no expectation of anything in return. Loving all things with full detachment will support us on our path to Realization.

When we love our mind and body in this sense, we will take care of them and not neglect them. They exist by the grace of Nature. When we recognize the mind and body as connected to the Divine, and not as a possession we own, we will take care of them and remain detached at the same time. We will take care of them in a balanced fashion; we will not become obsessed with attending to them. In such a way, we should love everyone, live a simple life, and do our duties with full commitment while remaining detached. This is what is meant when the sages say, "Live like a drop of water on a lotus leaf."

CHAPTER SIX

MANY PATHS, ONE GOAL

बहवः पन्थानः

In the city of Mysore, India, there is a bus stand where twenty or thirty buses line up at any given time awaiting departure to cities all over India. People who want to find a bus for the city of Bangalore will often approach the conductor and ask, "Is this Bangalore?" Of course, that bus is not actually the *city* of Bangalore. But the bus is a vehicle that travels to Bangalore, so when the conductor says, "Yes," people board that bus and take a seat with some assurance that they will eventually arrive in Bangalore!

The direct meaning of the word *yoga* is Samādhi—the union of the Self with the Eternal Truth. There are many paths that can lead us to this experience. These paths are also called yoga, but only in the secondary sense. Like the bus to Bangalore, they only help carry us to the final destination, which itself is Samādhi, or Realization. Only if the path leads to this supreme human experience should one consider it yoga; otherwise, it has been misnamed. If our desired destination is the yogic experience, we should question the available paths or techniques by asking, "Is this yoga?" The answer must be, "Only if the technique is used as a vehicle to reach the final destination itself, Samādhi."

THREE PATHS LEADING HOME

Imagine we enter a wilderness area to hike and enjoy the beautiful views, or search for flowers and precious herbs. While wandering in these surroundings, we become disoriented and eventually lost. Our desire is to return home, where everything is familiar and comfortable, but how do we find our way back? From a yogic perspective, there are three main approaches to solve our dilemma.

First, if we possess a very good memory, we can simply pause and recollect the route by which we came. We think about the lay of the land and note the various rivers and ponds we passed along the way, we recall the hills and valleys we crossed, and gradually we retrace our steps. The clarity of our memory is what gives us the confidence needed to find our way home again.

Second, if we happen to meet someone who is familiar with this area and knows the location of our village, he can provide us with a map and a set of instructions. Understanding the area, he will suggest a suitable route and advise us on what we might encounter along our way. He may even teach us various skills for traveling in the wilderness. If we follow those instructions, step by step, we will reach our home safely through our own human effort. The only requirement is that we proceed diligently, and that our efforts remain sincere and persistent, until we reach our home.

Third, if we happen to meet someone who is traveling in the direction of our home, we can simply follow along. If this person is a frequent traveler in these parts, he will know the route very well. With so much knowledge, he is capable of helping us in many ways. Through the grace of Nature, he may be compassionate and sympathetic and have our welfare at heart. Simply by following him, at some point, we will reach our home. Thus, we only need to attach ourselves to this person.

The methods described here are analogous to the three main paths in yoga. These are respectively, *Jñāna Yoga*, *Karma Yoga,* and *Bhakti Yoga*.

Jñāna Yoga is for a practitioner who already has most of the prerequisites for Realization by birth. This type of person is by nature detached. She will have a very good memory, a sharp intellect, and a high capacity for concentration. She will be naturally quiet and meditative. Because she possesses less preconditioning, she will be able to objectively see the nature of her mind. She will be able to identify the "I" and contemplate it. This is Jñāna Yoga, a path which requires a pure mind and a meditative mood. Subpaths of Jñāna Yoga include *Rāja Yoga* and *Laya Yoga* (see appendix).

Karma Yoga is for a practitioner with a lot of energy and capacity for work. As the knowledgeable man in the wilderness advises the lost wanderer about what to look for, and which skills to use on his homeward journey, the teacher of Karma Yoga will explain the right actions necessary for success on the yogic path. The student will receive practices and disciplines that correct imbalances in his mind and body so that he can gain yogic experiences. Subpaths of Karma Yoga include *Haṭha Yoga* and *Aṣṭāṅga Yoga,* among others.

Bhakti Yoga is for practitioners who naturally have more attachment tendencies. It is their nature to get attached to worldly things. Therefore, they need to use this tendency as their guide for Realization. This yogic path will primarily consist of attaching oneself to someone, or something, that can carry one to the final destination. This is the primary focus. When one finds a suitable object of attachment, one will gradually reach her goal. Subpaths of Bhakti Yoga will often include *Mantra Yoga, Japa Yoga,* and *Pūja Yoga*—in which devotion is the main focus of the path. In total, there are nine additional types of devotional subpaths of Bhakti Yoga, which include *Śravaṇa Bhakti* and *Smaraṇa Bhakti*.

Jñāna Yoga, Karma Yoga, and Bhakti Yoga are not mutually exclusive. All practitioners will use aspects of each of them, but one will be established as the primary route for an individual's practice. Even if a practitioner is a jñāna yogi, devotion and right action will still be necessary for progress. If a practitioner is naturally a karma yogi, he will still need a good intellect and the capacity to cultivate proper devotion and attachment to the Divine. Likewise, a bhakti yogi requires some aspects of the other two paths, as well.

Any valid yogic path can be classified into one of these three primary paths. And, within each primary path, there are thousands of subpaths. All aim to correct the mind and body. By sincerely following any one, the practitioner will receive great benefits to help her achieve final Liberation.

JÑĀNA YOGA: AN INQUIRY INTO THE SELF

Artists sometimes draw pictures that cleverly merge two images. At first glance, most people will see only one or the other image. For example, we might initially see a forest and some rivers. Then, if we relax our vision and redirect our focus a little, we suddenly see the entire image actually forms the shape of an elephant. The rivers we initially saw actually make up the elephant's trunk and tail and the forest and mountains become the elephant's head and back. We then discover that by simply shifting our gaze, we are able to see both images.

Oceanographers have discovered fish in the ocean that skillfully camouflage themselves. A scientist may show us a photo of these fish resting on the ocean floor, and all we see is sand, coral, and stones. Only when the scientist points out various features of the fish do we suddenly recognize it as a fish and marvel at its clever deception.

Actually, the mind resembles such images. It takes an experienced yogi to teach a student how to properly view its multiple dimensions. The mind contains impressions of this external world, as well as of the Eternal Truth. The yogi will suggest to the student which of these impressions—arising thoughts and images—to concentrate upon and which to ignore and try to forget. At some point, the student will be able to grasp the Eternal Truth alone and thereby become Realized.

This is Jñāna Yoga, a path that suits a highly sattvic personality. *Jñāna* translates in Saṃskṛta as "knowledge"; however, the original meaning is Eternal Truth.

Jñāna Yoga requires us to deeply and analytically understand the mind. The practitioner then aims to reduce the mind's activity and modifications and remove all preconditioning. Eventually he will begin to experience bliss or light, or both. He will follow this until he gradually forgets the whole world and visualizes the Eternal Truth.

There are many references to the ṛṣi Yājñavalkya in the Upaniṣads, the sacred literature of the sages. He was a jñāna yogi. Because of a keen intellect, clear perception, pure mind, healthy body, and the absence of preconditioning, yogis like Yājñavalkya were able to discern the evidence of the Eternal Truth in their minds. They easily understood the deep meaning behind the question, Who is the "I"?

Ramana Maharshi is a recent example of one who applied this practice of Jñāna Yoga. As a small boy, he was naturally detached from the external world. He had a serious quest for knowledge, asking, "Who am I?" This question compelled him to leave his childhood home and go into solitude to meditate for years. He sat in such deep inquiry on the nature of the Self that he was completely unaware of the ants and insects that would come and bite his body. Because of his dedication, he achieved Realization. His example inspired many others on this path.

Like Ramana Maharshi, a practitioner on this path develops an intense interest for Realization and is capable of becoming completely detached from worldly affairs. When that is combined with a strong discipline to contemplate on the Self, it may be possible to achieve Liberation on one's own. When this occurs, one will be guided by the Eternal Truth itself—the teacher of all teachers. However, even when one's constitution is right for this path, it is nearly impossible without some guidance. The best guidance will come from a Realized teacher.

An aspirant may come to live at such a teacher's āśrama in order to receive direction. Living near the teacher, attending to daily duties, and studying various teachings all serve a central purpose: to be close to a Realized Soul and to observe the way she lives. Through watching the teacher on a daily basis, the student uncovers clues to and guidance on what constitutes an ideal lifestyle. This experience has a more profound impact than simply hearing words: The teaching finds its way to the heart of the student. He will develop an accurate understanding of the universe, and this will gradually give rise to a balanced mind and body. This is the kind of maturity a true teacher inspires.

A teacher will wait many years for the student to mature. At some point, she will feel a great flood of tenderness and compassion as an indication that it is time to lead the student further. The teacher will explain the bliss of Samādhi and portray a vivid picture of the bright light, divine sound, and bliss of the Eternal Truth. This image will inspire a quest for further knowledge in the depths of the student's heart. Then the teacher will reveal the hidden Truth: *"Tatvamasi,"* meaning, "You are the Soul. You are the Eternal Truth." Coming directly from the experience of a Realized Soul, these words will have the power to convey their exact meaning. A mature student needs no other technique than contemplation. When a Realized person encourages a mature student to contemplate directly on "I," the mature student will forget everything except this "I" and will attain Realization. No other techniques are required. This is how a few words from a Realized person can lead to Realization. And because the student is ready to hear them, he will receive them deep within his heart and begin to meditate on them. He may then begin to experience a divine light, sound, or bliss. Gradually, he will forget the whole world, realize the Self, and visualize the Eternal Truth. Thus, he will become Liberated. This is how a true teacher instructs using the path of Jñāna Yoga.

KARMA YOGA: A JOURNEY TO INNER LIGHT

In the beginning of this chapter, we discussed how we become lost in the forest of the external world. The reason for our predicament lies within our actions, or karma. We have entered the forest, and now additional action is required to remedy our situation. Just as a knowledgeable and compassionate person can advise a lost wanderer on how to return home, the path of Karma Yoga can guide us with the right actions necessary to reach our final goal. Thus, Karma Yoga is the yoga of *right action*.

Our bodies are made for action. If we do not perform actions, we cannot exist. However, because we sometimes engage in inappropriate actions and behaviors, imbalances occur in our system. Nature will attempt to correct these errors through intervening divine energies present both inside and outside our bodies. For example, if one is overstrained, his system will make him sleepy; if he takes rest and sleeps, his system will be corrected. If we accept Nature's corrections, we can eliminate many of our problems. But due to māyā's influence, we are often unable to fully grasp the hidden messages Nature provides. Thus, we require some guidance.

The practice of Karma Yoga requires us to understand right action and then to engage in it for an extended period of time. The key is to engage in right actions without being attached to them or their results. If we do this, day by day our body will come to a natural condition of health and balance. Gradually, we will gain this health because we are living according to the divine principles of Nature. When our actions are in harmony with our system, many of our previous errors—from this life, as well as past lives—are eliminated. When they are sufficiently reduced, we will have fewer thoughts and modifications of mind that lead us away from the causal state of pradāna. Our tendency for future error will be greatly limited. This is how the practice of Karma Yoga brings a practitioner to gradually experience Samādhi. Both Haṭha Yoga and Aṣṭāṅga Yoga are considered subpaths of Karma Yoga because the role of human effort and action underlie their various disciplines.

BHAKTI YOGA: THE PATH OF DEVOTION

Many people have a tendency toward deep attachment. This tendency binds them to the cycle of birth and death. Through ignorance, they become attached to some worldly object or material, such as money, power, sensual pleasures, and the like. These are all powerful hooks that ensnare us and only develop further cravings and attachments. Fortunately, our tendency for attachment can itself be used for Liberation. For this to occur, however, we must substitute these familiar objects of attachment with those associated with the Eternal Truth. This is Bhakti Yoga, the path of devotion.

What we become attached to can either cause misery or support us in our quest for Liberation. Eternal Truth exists everywhere in the universe—in human beings, other animals, birds, insects, water, air, rock, earth, sun, moon, and stars. However, some material objects are closer to the Eternal Truth than others. This is because they possess a predominance of sattvic energy in their constitutions. A qualified teacher may assign such an object to a student for devotion. This may be an image of a deity or teacher, a particular chant, or some other sattvic aspect of nature. When the student becomes sincerely devoted to this object, he will gradually visualize the Eternal Truth.

As in this chapter's opening story, we enter into the forest because of external cravings and attachments—to enjoy the beautiful views or to search for flowers and precious herbs. However, we find our way home through our attachment to our guide and his teachings. Bhakti Yoga encourages us to convert our attachment tendencies into devotion to find our way to the Divine, our true home. The great sages say, "Use this very attachment that has caught you to free yourself from its grip. Simply change your direction and attach yourself to some divine object that is nearer to the Eternal Truth, and it will then become your link to it."

BEST PATH = NEAREST PATH

Imagine the universe is a great tree with three main branches representing the three main branches of yoga—Jñāna Yoga, Karma Yoga, and Bhakti Yoga. Every person sits on one of these three branches. If the Eternal Truth is the root of the tree, each person must use her branch to move, first to the trunk, and then the root. We cannot begin from someone else's starting point. Some will sit closer to the trunk and therefore have an easier experience reaching the root, the Eternal Truth. Where each person begins will determine which of the three main yogic paths she will use to reach the final goal. Therefore, one's path and experience on that path will be largely determined by one's own individual karma and *constitution*. Thus, the best yogic path for an individual is the yogic path nearest to that individual.

INDIVIDUAL CONSTITUTION

The best yoga path for any one of us is determined by our *physical constitution*. This is based on the three fundamental body components, or *doṣas,* known as *vāta, pitta,* and *kapha*. Each doṣa embodies a different combination of the five basic elements: *space, air, fire, water,* and *earth*. Each of us will contain some combination of all three doṣas. We will generally have a single doṣa or, more commonly, a combination of two that predominate in our system. In rare cases, all three may be equally present. Human beings can be categorized into seven physical constitutional types. In addition to the three primary constitutions (vāta, pitta, kapha), there are four additional combinations (vāta-pitta, vāta-kapha, pitta-kapha, and vāta-pitta-kapha).

A person's constitution is reflected in how he engages his mind and body. A person of *vāta* constitution may constantly engage in physical activities and be inclined to work very hard. A person of *pitta* constitution is often dissatisfied unless he is engaged intellectually. A person of *kapha* constitution is not generally attracted to strenuous physical or mental work; he would rather keep his mind in a reflective mood. He just wants to be happy and to enjoy calmness and quietness.

Other individual factors, such as maturity, saṃskāras, the historical times in which we live, and, of course, our own human effort, can greatly influence our constitutions. This can be seen when two people share the same constitution. For example, two scientists are both pitta dominant. They are both sitting on the same branch of the tree, but one is honest, and the other is deceitful. One eats wholesome foods and has a healthy, strong mind and body, while the other eats a poor diet and is obese and sickly. One attends to his duties promptly, but the other shirks his responsibilities. This wide diversity within a single constitution reflects the other influencing factors, which determine how a particular constitution may manifest in a person's life. Many individuals share some constitutional makeup or combination of doṣas, but depending on their previous actions and births, they will be inclined to take different actions in this lifetime. Some people may be innately honest, whereas others will need to cultivate honesty. In the same way, some will be inherently trusting, while others will be suspicious of everyone around them. Some will be attached and addicted to objects and materials; others will be less attached; and a few will be born with no attachment at all. These attachments reflect imbalances, or saṃskāras, that a person needs to correct and is the basic reason that we find so many types of characters, behaviors, mentalities, and tendencies in human beings.

Each person will prepare for taking a trip based on the destination and the length of his visit. A person traveling to a nearby city and returning the same day will take his wallet and perhaps a lunch. A person leaving for a business trip will pack a small suitcase with several changes of clothes, some personal items, and perhaps some needed medications. A person leaving for a trip around the world will make more elaborate preparations; along with clothes for varied weather conditions, he may take a favorite book or two, perhaps a few items he uses for hobbies in his leisure time, photos of his family, various maps, and so on.

In a similar way, we are taking a journey back to our original "home," the Self. Our starting point along this journey is based on our previous births' saṃskāra. Someone who is close to the Eternal Truth has already developed many of the skills and much of the knowledge she requires to complete her journey. A person farther away lacks some of these necessities.

LIMBS OF A PATH

Having chosen a yogic path, an aspirant must then understand which disciplines and practices to follow to reach the final goal. The individual disciplines and practices are the limbs of a given path. Within each limb there resides one or more disciplines or techniques to master that limb. These, too, will be determined by our individual needs, maturity, saṃskāras, the times in which we live, and our own human effort.

How does a seeker decide which yogic path or limbs to practice? Customarily, a knowledgeable teacher will determine this. He will be able to see both the strengths and weaknesses of a student. He will choose the appropriate path based on the student's constitution. He will also be able to see which yogic limbs are already inherent in the student and which are absent. Such a teacher will then direct the student by recommending specific yogic limbs through a particular yogic path to correct the student's system.

WHAT IS MOST ESSENTIAL?

The particular yoga path one chooses, and the number of limbs one practices within that path, will vary from person to person. There may be two, four, eight, fifteen, or even more limbs to a given path. For example, Rāja Yoga contains two; Haṭha Yoga is delineated into four; Aṣṭāṅga Yoga into eight; and *Pañcādaśāṅga Yoga,* a path similar to Aṣṭāṅga Yoga, divides the practice into fifteen. For a few, however, yoga will consist of only one limb: Samādhi. This is because fewer external practices are required for them to naturally experience a yogic state.

However, there is a powerful link between the eight limbs of Aṣṭāṅga Yoga and Realization. This is because the goal of Realization can be more easily achieved by developing these eight important disciplines within our system. While all the various yogic paths will inherently include aspects of these eight limbs, Aṣṭāṅga Yoga presents clear guidelines and disciplines for beginners on the yogic journey. These eight limbs will help the student to perfect these disciplines.

PART TWO

AṢṬĀṄGA YOGA

Yamas & Niyamas

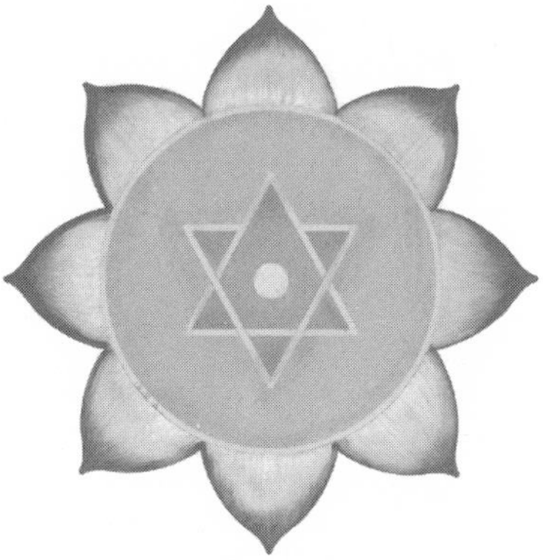

IN THIS SECTION we will try to understand the most popular yoga path in the world today—Aṣṭāṅga Yoga, the eight limbs of yoga. To clarify, we are referring in this book to the ancient eight-limbed Aṣṭāṅga Yoga path and not only the rigorous asana sequences, also referred to as aṣṭāṅga yoga. The greatness of this path is that it can be practiced by anyone, regardless of one's constitution. This is because it includes the most essential disciplines and practices an aspirant needs to reach the final goal and experience the Eternal Truth. From the first steps to the final goal, this path guides a practitioner to develop a disciplined life, an ideal *yogic way of life*. Beginning with any one of the eight limbs (or many sub-limbs), a practitioner will easily develop the necessary confidence to master the remaining limbs.

A STURDY VEHICLE OF EIGHT LIMBS

In Saṃskṛta, *aṣṭa* means "eight"; *aṅga* means "limb." Aṣṭāṅga Yoga is a path with eight limbs: yama, niyama, āsana, prāṇāyāma, pratyāhāra, dhāraṇā, dhyāna, and Samādhi.

The *yamas* offer a set of disciplines that mainly help us control our five senses and five organs of action. *Niyamas* offer a set of disciplines that mainly help us control our mind. Āsana focuses on the postures that help us steady our body and keep it comfortable for long periods of time. *Prāṇāyāma* brings control over our breath and reduces our mind's activity. *Pratyāhāra* cultivates withdrawal of our senses from external objects. While *dhāraṇā* is a concentration technique that allows our mind to focus on a single object, through *dhyāna* we maintain *uninterrupted* focus on a single object; dhyāna leads to the last limb, of Samādhi. In this context we mean *Samprajñāta Samādhi,* the *practice* of Samādhi. The actual *final goal,* the ultimate aim of the previous eight limbs, is *Asamprajñāta Samādhi.* Finally, within each limb, there are sub-limbs. For instance, *ahimsā,* "nonviolence," and *satya,* "truthfulness," are sub-limbs of the yama limb.

On the yogic path, the limbs are like those of our body. If we want to walk to the next town, all limbs of our body must cooperate. Our feet cannot go to the next town while leaving our hands behind. In yoga, all limbs must cooperate to take us to the final destination.

For example, a farmer may wish to grow a perfect apple with many fine qualities. It should be sweet and juicy, as well as have a beautiful color and attractive fragrance. In naturally developed fruit, all attributes will usually develop together. Nature will rarely manifest one characteristic without the others. If the farmer wants to develop one of these qualities fully, all the others, ideally, will be present to some degree. For the apple to have a beautiful color and shape, it will also likely be sweet and juicy. Contrary to Nature, today's artificial hybridization and genetic modification of plants and animals often enhance only one or two qualities while degrading others.

An important distinction is that limbs are not *steps*. If they were steps, we would take them sequentially. But because they are like the limbs of our body, they need to work together. If our aim is to recondition our mind and body to its original state, we need to develop capacities in all eight limbs. We would think it humorous if a man went to a health club and decided to make his right arm strong while ignoring his left.

It is also true that if any limb or sub-limb of yoga is established absolutely, all the remaining limbs will automatically be found to some extent. It is impossible to have one limb in perfect form and any of the remaining totally absent.

For example, the Aṣṭāṅga Yoga limb āsana, requires sitting in a stable, comfortable posture without movement or strain for a long period. If the practitioner has an unconditioned mind that is calm and not misguided by preconceptions and expectations, he will identify what disturbs him while sitting; he will understand if his body needs some correction, and he might include a second āsana to make that correction. If the practitioner has told a lie, that lie will disturb his sitting practice, and he will be compelled toward more truthfulness in his future behavior. If he has eaten too much, that will disturb his practice, and he will understand he needs to correct his eating habits. As a result of his clear and calm mind, he will identify and bring all other limbs and sub-limbs of yoga to the right condition, one by one, consciously or unconsciously. Thus, although one limb may be primary, our aim should be to develop all limbs at the same time.

THE POWER OF YOGIC LIMBS

The yogic scriptures make many bold statements regarding the power of the various limbs of yoga: Telling the absolute truth establishes a yogi in the Eternal Truth; if nonviolence is practiced to the fullest extent, one will realize God; if one āsana, *siddhāsana,* is mastered, then everything is achieved. The underlying principle is that when we finally follow any one discipline, this corrects all aspects of the personality required for Realization. We are able to visualize the Divine through any limb. Because of this, there are thousands of methods to achieve Liberation. They are all known as yogic paths. If we journey through ancient times, we come across many instances of yogis achieving Realization through one or another such practice.

In very rare cases a human being will be naturally born manifesting perfection of all limbs of yoga. Her mind and body will be healthy and strong. She will easily feel detached from the material world. She will be content and happy in her life. She will perform her duty promptly without fail. Possessing all these requirements, she would have a balanced mentality that would enable her to quickly achieve Realization. She would need only a small reminder from a knowledgeable teacher, or from Nature itself, to realize the Self and become Liberated.

For all human beings, regardless of their individual constitution, karma, and saṃskāra, Nature has provided a path with which they may reach the final goal. It is important we find such a suitable path—preferably through a knowledgeable teacher—and stick with it rather than jumping from one path to another. For a person seeking water, better to dig one well sixty feet deep than to dig ten wells each only six feet deep! Within each yogic path, the various limbs make a whole and healthy human being. When we nurture all the limbs and are in good condition, we become human beings with great capacities. When we use our full potential with sincere effort, we can make our way to Realization and Liberation.

Aṣṭāṅga Yoga tames the system from many different angles. For example, our three tools of *mind*, *speech*, and *body* may be used to commit many errors in life that lead to attachment and suffering. Through the various practices and disciplines outlined in this path, these three tools will come into balance and become powerful agents on our path toward Liberation.

Though Aṣṭāṅga Yoga is classified as a subpath of Karma Yoga, it is one of the most important yogic paths in all of yoga. The great sage Yājñavalkya has said, "The Realization of Self is yoga that is endowed with eight limbs." As we have said, Realization may be attained following any yogic path; however, the eight limbs of Aṣṭāṅga Yoga will play a role in all of them. Unless we acquire some minimal control over our five senses and our mind through the yamas and niyamas; establish stillness in our body and posture through āsana; control our breath through prāṇāyāma; withdraw the mind from the external world through pratyāhāra; focus our contemplation on one object through dhāraṇā; obtain uninterrupted one-objectedness of the mind through dhyāna; and forget all our human effort in this whole process through Samādhi, Realization is impossible.

Some level of effort is required to correct any disturbance found within our human systems. This effort is nothing but karma. This is why Aṣṭāṅga Yoga is considered as Karma Yoga. Through proper study, one will come to understand that these two yogas are basically one and the same. This oneness is implied by the fact that the eight limbs offer a path toward living an ideal life, and this ideal life is a result of ideal action in the world.

In the Bhagavad-Gītā, one of the most widely honored yogic texts which contains the very core of yoga philosophy, we are presented with a vivid account and description of Karma Yoga. In the text *Yogi Yājñavalkya,* another classical yogic text, the sage Yājñavalkya describes an equally vivid description of Aṣṭāṅga Yoga. In both of these texts, right action, or ideal action, is the most important factor.

Let us bow our head to the great sage Patañjali, known as an incarnation of Kuṇḍalinī, who systematically and eloquently presented to us the Yoga Sūtras, the second chapter of which offers us the core principles of Aṣṭāṅga Yoga. Here we get a glimpse of the richness and benefits of the Aṣṭāṅga Yoga path. It is our primary aim in the following chapters to expand upon these wonderful teachings.

CHAPTER SEVEN

THE YAMAS

महाव्रतम्

THE EIGHT LIMBS of Aṣṭāṅga Yoga lead an aspirant on a path from the external to the internal, where the Eternal Truth resides. From the external standpoint, the yamas are the most important limb.

In *Yogi Yājñavalkya,* Yājñavalkya describes ten yamas. In the Yoga Sūtras, Patañjali combines several of these and describes only five—the more common number discussed today. For example, Patañjali's description of nonviolence, or ahimsā, includes Yājñavalkya's notion of *mitāhāra*, or right food, as well as his notion of *kṣamā*, or tolerance. Likewise, Yājñavalkya's *ārjava,* or straightforwardness, is included in Patañjali's concept of satya, or truthfulness.

There are no fundamental differences of opinion between Patañjali and Yājñavalkya; rather, they simply use slightly different terminology and styles to convey their ideas. Patañjali uses *aphorisms,* a style that is more succinct and precise. He carefully chooses each word to communicate broad concepts. Yājñavalkya, however, explains each idea in detail. For this book, we have selected his ten yamas: *ahimsā, satya, asteya, brahmacarya, aparigraha, dayā, ārjava, kṣamā, dhṛti,* and *mitāhāra*. One need not worry whether there are five, ten, twelve, or some other number; our aim is simply to understand the heart of the sages' message.

AHIMSĀ: NONVIOLENCE

When I was sixteen years old, I was studying in high school and living in the village where I was born. My family owned a beautiful farm, and I often worked alongside the hired laborers. I was enthusiastic, industrious, and watchful by nature. One day I was walking in the fields alongside an elderly woman of about seventy years, whom my father had hired. I remember her name was Addu. We were collecting

Āyurvedic herbs. I held a machete-like tool that I had made myself, sharpening the edge with a stone. As we walked down the path together, I saw a small tree-like plant three or four feet high. Suddenly, I had an urge to test the sharpness of my tool. With one swing I cut the plant from its roots. Addu saw what I had done and said, "Oh, sir, you should never do like this. These plants are like children. They, too, are having life."

I was stunned and embarrassed. Later, when we were about to collect a small plant for medicinal purposes, she expressed her gratitude and compassion for that plant, saying, "Never should we harm anything unnecessarily."

I was from a well-educated Brahmin family, while Addu was an uneducated laborer. Yet she spoke with such compassion and tenderness that her words went straight to my heart. This simple woman was imparting profound knowledge about the first yama: *ahimsā*, or *nonviolence*. This kind of understanding cannot come through formal education. It made me think deeply and taught me a lesson that I will remember my whole life. Today, whenever I see this particular plant growing somewhere, I think of this incident.

Truth, *sacredness*, and *beauty* are the three most important characteristics seen throughout this universe. They come from the Eternal Truth and are contained in everything to a greater or lesser extent. Happiness takes shelter under their protection. In yogic literature, these three are known as *satyam, śivam,* and *sundaram.* Violence can utterly spoil them. When we intentionally violate these qualities, we violate Truth. It is therefore our duty to preserve and maintain them. This is what underlies ahimsā. Patañjali lists it as the first yama, and it is considered the most important.

THREE FORMS OF VIOLENCE

There are three basic forms of violence. The first occurs through physically maltreating another. The second form is verbal, or the violence that arises from our words. The third form of violence occurs through the power of our thoughts.

Physical violence is the grossest form of violence. War, rage, and anger may all lead individuals to lash out physically at one another.

Intentionally harming another person physically carries with it tremendous energy and negative karma. This kind of violence lodges deeply in the mind and body, causing disturbances not only for the victim, but also for the perpetrator and witnesses. All sentient beings in the universe have the right to live. They all want a calm and quiet life, to whatever extent their nature will allow. If we go against this, Nature will reprimand us. Disturbances caused by violence agitate the mind and become an enormous hindrance to the yogic experience.

The second form of violence is verbal. We can cause many types of injury through what we say. Whatever we utter, whether it is with good intentions or not, can cause disturbances. If we say something that is not agreeable to other people, we can disturb their minds. The ability to talk is a gift of Nature. If we use this gift to hurt someone else, we are committing violence.

Words alone can cause severe disturbances. This is because words not only carry an idea from one person to another; they can also convey a type of commanding energy. Sometimes this energy carries tremendous power and may inflict a wound in the form of psychological damage, or may even cause death. This is what underlies a *curse.* A curse should not be confused with simply insulting or swearing at another. Verbally cursing someone can lead to serious negative conditions. A person may even die as a result of a curse. A few possess this power of the tongue from birth; others may gain this ability through an intense practice of truthfulness.

When we communicate something to another, we must try to do so in a way that does no harm. Our words must never be unduly harsh, even when our intention is honorable. There are various methods of expression, and we need to know how to express our message so as not to hurt anybody. Sometimes a situation may arise in which it becomes our duty to correct some imbalance or disturbance caused by others. If faced with this situation, we may have to use words that hurt, but only as a last resort. Even then, we must choose our words carefully, because they will cause disturbances on both sides. Overall, this disturbance should be less injurious than the initial imbalance.

The third type of violence is through the power of the mind. To a lesser or greater extent, each individual possesses this power. It may be acquired or inherent. Regardless of its origin, it will have an influence on others. Violence occurs when this power is used to wish someone harm. When we wish someone harm, it is a form of cursing. It disturbs another according to the power of the person's mind who curses and the vulnerability of the one being cursed. According to the relative power of the curse and the vulnerability of the one being cursed, it can cause significant disturbance.

Two kinds of disturbances arise for the person who curses. The first is direct. When we wish something bad for others, we will become agitated immediately, due to our menacing thoughts. The second is indirect, more like an echo. When we wish something bad for another, the turmoil they suffer will come back in some indirect way to affect us. If they do not suffer, then we will be left with karma that must take its own course. Our faulty thought process causes all these unwanted disturbances.

Why would we want to disturb ourselves by harming someone else? Instead of cursing others, we can help ourselves tremendously if we bless them. This will greatly benefit others as well as ourselves. The power of our goodwill and sincere intention will build our internal capacity. Instead of causing psychological or physical disturbances to others, we heal our own psychic wounds. This is one way to make our minds more fit and balanced in order to practice yoga.

THREE METHODS OF VIOLENCE

In addition to these three basic forms of violence, there are three *methods* by which we can inflict this violence upon others. The first involves direct, personal injury to someone else, using our body, words, or mind. Second, we can provoke another to violence. For example, if a manager or boss provokes a subordinate to violence, he has indirectly perpetrated that violence. The third method involves our direct or indirect approval. For instance, if we condone some sort of violence in the world, directly or indirectly, then we ourselves have contributed to it. Any direct or indirect approval of violence encourages violent tendencies. All these methods of inflicting violence not only disturb our psychology and physiology, but form karma that in turn will gain momentum and lead us to further acts of violence.

To maintain harmony, we are often advised to remain silent. There are times, however, when silence may indirectly cause harm. For instance, it is considered a form of violence for a person to keep quiet when aware of someone else's intention or act of committing a crime that harms other people. In such cases, one should reveal the truth to the proper authorities. This is considered our duty.

Although yogis wholeheartedly recommend nonviolence, they are aware that total nonviolence is not possible in this world. There are times when violence is unavoidable and even accepted by Nature. When we harvest food to eat, we commit violence. When we walk, talk, or even inhale and exhale, we kill insects and other microscopic life forms. Yet life is based on these activities. We cannot live without walking, talking, eating, and breathing. What is the remedy for these infringements? We must try, at all times, to minimize the violence that we commit. One way to do this is by taking only necessary actions. Another is to ask the forgiveness of Nature. In addition, we need to have mercy for those we hurt. Finally, if we achieve Realization, those insects that we have killed directly or indirectly will be benefited because their lives served our path toward Realization.

This is one more reason that Realization is the best possible goal for human life. In every action, there is a measure of violence. If we dedicate all actions, taken directly or indirectly, to the purposes of Realization, only then can we avoid the repercussions of violence. If we engage in violence because of egotism, and without mercy, we will create a violent karma, causing disturbance in our current life, and carrying saṃskāras into the next one.

In a deeper sense, since all actions cause violence, the wise will walk only when it is required, speak only when it is most essential, and consume no more than what is necessary. This contradicts the pattern that we see in the modern world today, where society demands more travel and constant communication by computers and cell phones. In addition, there is far too little support for moderation in the consumption of food and other resources.

We think that abundant consumption symbolizes prosperity, but we do not understand its hidden problems. People get caught up in this rat race, and it generates cravings for more and more material goods.

For example, after watching a TV commercial, a man yearns to own a luxury automobile. He then takes out a large loan to pay for it and spends six years paying it back. Sixty seconds of delusion causes six years of suffering!

In the early part of the twentieth century in India, this tendency of overconsumption was not so prevalent. Many people had only two sets of clothing. Each day, one set would be worn while the other was being laundered. If an average person wore simple clothes, it did not reduce his or her prestige. On the contrary, the villagers would honor one another for living in harmony with nature. Today this tendency is gradually being lost, and even people in the villages are beginning to crave more material objects.

Since all actions are associated with some violence, once we have begun an activity, it is our duty to complete it. If we do not complete what we have started, we have wasted effort and caused some meaningless violence. If we are judicious, we will begin as few activities as possible, and only those that are essential. We should think twice about collecting experiences and accomplishments simply to add to our name and fame. Each of these will come with some karmic consequences. Most people will not think of this unless they seriously contemplate the cause-and-consequence principle. If we reduce our activities to the minimum, we will reduce the consequences associated with their karma.

EATING FOOD

Eating is an unavoidable form of violence. We must take nourishment from sources that are living or that were once alive. But we often eat more than is necessary for optimal health. Eating only what we require ensures that our body is proportionate, healthy, clean, and light. More important is this principle: Starting at birth, nature allots us a certain amount of food to eat; when we have consumed our allotment, we die and move on to the next stage in our evolution.

In Saṃskṛta, the word for food is *annam*. The sacred Upaniṣad scriptures explain, "You are eating the food, and at the same time it is eating you." There are three reasons for this. First, the body undergoes undue strain while digesting overgenerous portions of food. Second, the energy that we collect from this food stirs and provokes our system to be overactive, and this again creates strain. Third, Nature has provided a certain amount of food for us, and if we eat more than that, we are eating food that is meant for others, and this will have an adverse effect. Eating even one more mouthful of food than we require begins to rob the food that we have consumed of its nourishing effects. It becomes detrimental to the body, thereby decreasing our lifespan. Eating less will allow us to enjoy a healthy body longer. Most important, the combination of a healthy body and a long life affords us the best possible opportunity to practice yoga and move toward Realization.

Almost without exception, the eating habits of people who live in rural villages in India are appropriate for their energy expenditure, primarily because they are not burdened with much stress and strain. They enjoy a peaceful way of life. By contrast, people in cities are busy from morning to evening, and this excessive busyness causes stress. Many people all around the world overeat because of the stress and strain in their lives.

Attempting to control what we eat while failing to address the root cause of overeating is futile. This problem cannot be conquered through a direct frontal attack. Such an attack will simply provoke the problem to take a new form. We cannot control this habit unless we find a calm and quiet way of life. We need to stop chasing after material phantoms that masquerade as happiness. When we cannot adequately fulfill those cravings, we often turn to eating. However, by realigning our way of life with yogic principles, problems with overeating may be resolved naturally and gracefully. If we have a balanced approach toward material possessions, live calmly, and focus on a proper spiritual target for our life, we will be more easily satisfied overall. The amount we eat will easily and naturally decrease. Moreover, a contented person will eat less. As we begin to enjoy the results of our practice, and savor the happiness that comes from the core of our heart through yoga, we will eat less.

THE AMOUNT OF FOOD TO EAT

There is much to understand about the amount of food we need to eat. We must acquire an objective view about our own body and the activity necessary to perform our duties. If we are doing very strenuous physical work, we need to eat sufficient food to sustain our bodies in that work. But generally, yogis observe that most of us eat far more food than is physiologically required.

This statement is true from two standpoints. First, we do many activities that are contrary to nature or are unnecessary to begin with. These activities do not contribute to our happiness. They do not help us in our progress toward Realization. In fact, many of them disturb us and hinder our yogic path. We are scurrying unnecessarily from here to there, and we conclude that we need a lot of energy because we feel depleted, and so we overeat.

Second, many people eat to satisfy the tongue rather than to fulfill the needs of the body, so that what they eat does not nourish them. Many people do not understand the real needs of the body. They have not cultivated the practice of eating with the goal of nourishing the body. Even though someone is eating too much, he also may be suffering from physical weakness due to malnutrition.

Our body will generally stay in the best condition if we eat small quantities of *sattvic* food that is easily digested, nonstimulating, and calming to the mind and body. In addition, we should engage in a mild level of physical activity. If we participate in more moderate physical activities, we must slightly increase our intake. However, we will disturb our system if we eat more than we are able to burn off through our physical activity. Eating energizes our system, and it will provoke the mind or body. Too much provocation disturbs the mind and spurs the body to be active or want to work hard. If we do not find a way to release this excess energy, we accumulate body fat. The use of sattvic food commensurate with our level of activity will never harm us.

Some people feel shaky and unwell if they miss a meal by a few hours. The primary cause is often that they are consuming incorrect foods. The food may be unsuitable for their constitution, inappropriate for their current situation, or of incorrect proportion. Eating incorrect foods brings imbalance to the mind and body, limiting our ability to assess our system. If we eat the correct amount of healthy food, and we follow this discipline consistently, we will gain the power of precise introspection and can use this power to increase our level of health.

VEGETARIANISM

Human beings have the option to eat meat or vegetables. All food, both vegetarian and nonvegetarian, is or was alive. Let us assume that to experience happiness implies some level of consciousness. Considering the ability to experience happiness as a gauge of life, we find that animals have a far greater capacity to experience it than vegetation. To destroy the ability to experience happiness is a serious act with karmic consequences. For this simple reason, eating vegetarian food is less violent than eating nonvegetarian food.

There are many reasons to avoid nonvegetarian foods. Today the methods used to raise animals are mostly inhumane. The animals live with no freedom in prison-like cages from birth to their last minute of life. They are fed against the laws of nature in ways that cause artificial growth and painful mutations to their bodies.

Dairies around the world today are often run like factories and at times in a very violent manner. Previously in India, milk was never sold. It was an honorable deed to offer it freely to those who needed it. Today, the dairyman's interest is often only on production, efficiency, and profit. The living conditions of his animals may be very poor. Cows are impregnated for the sole purpose of initiating lactation. Therefore, after a cow gives birth, the calf is immediately taken away. For the most part, male calves are killed or raised for meat. But the cow instinctively wants to feed her milk to the calf. She cannot speak a language intelligible to humans. If we watch her after the calf is taken away, she will cry. We can see tears in her eyes. As a result, the milk will contain her pain. The influence of such food on our mind and body is enormous. It leads to a variety of illnesses in our bodies and emotional troubles. Such food cannot help humankind in its quest for Liberation. On the contrary, it is a total hindrance.

Today some follow the principles of veganism—eating no dairy products or other foods that exploit animals in any way—proving that one may live a perfectly healthy life eating in such a manner. Yet yoga maintains that even eating vegetables is killing. It is violence, but we cannot live without eating, and we cannot achieve Realization without living. This is why yogic philosophy suggests that the primary purpose for eating should be for Realization. If we eat with this intention, the souls of the life forms that we consume will benefit because of their link to us when we reach that goal. However, we must still try and minimize the violence involved in eating. At the same time we should show gratitude to those beings that offer their lives for our welfare. It is then our duty to use the energy we receive from them to aid the welfare of other living beings.

Many years ago, farmers were raising and nourishing animals with love and compassion. Animals experienced much more freedom and happiness. Even methods used for killing animals were considered a kind of art, done with compassion and minimal pain. Commercialization and greed has caused the modern tragedy. Businesses are running after money, unaware of the tremendous violence of their dealings. Individuals who eat this nonvegetarian food also contribute both directly and indirectly to this violence.

On the other hand, if faced with starvation in the absence of vegetarian food, yoga allows that we may eat meat, but only as a last resort. There was once a great sage named Viśvāmitra, who found himself in this situation, so he had no choice but to eat the flesh of an animal. Later, he performed rituals and ceremonies to remove the adverse impact and continued his life with no further disturbance.

VIOLENCE AIMED AT OURSELVES

Previously, we discussed violence to others. But we also must avoid violence to ourselves. It is our duty to safeguard our bodies. Of course, problems may arise on our yogic path that cannot be removed without some discomfort, and the correction itself may be a form of violence. For example, if there is an impurity or imbalance in our body, we must eliminate it. Sometimes this is possible only through a rigorous discipline like fasting. This will strain the body, but unless the practitioner fasts, the impurities and toxins cannot be purged. This type of self-violence is sometimes essential, although only for as long as is necessary. It is accepted as a penance. Otherwise, our actions should never lead to harming our mind or body. We are obligated to protect both our mind and body with every means possible.

VIOLENT TENDENCIES

Because of a saṃskāra working in one's system, a person may not always be able to follow all the principles of nonviolence. In such a case, prior to inflicting violence, we must try to develop strong analytic reasoning to understand the consequences of our actions. This might include an analysis of whether this violence will affect many or just a few. The more we reflect prior to acting, the more we develop a capacity to withdraw our violent tendencies. Even if we are not able to eliminate violent tendencies completely, their intensity and consequences will be reduced. Such thoughts will create a new impression in the mind, and these will gain power over time. At some point, we will be able to overcome our violent tendencies completely.

The impact of violence on our surroundings and upon us is significant. Sometimes people will rationalize violence because they believe that the end justifies the means. They feel that because a certain worthy goal must be attained, it vindicates the use of violence. However, we need to understand that violence always has an impact. We must not forget or minimize this basic truth. In some cases, violence is truly necessary, but we must always search for a nonviolent alternative to meet our goals.

VIOLENCE THAT BENEFITS

A doctor will sometimes cause pain when treating his patients, but this a benevolent form of violence. Although it benefits the patient, it is violence, nevertheless. Āyurvedic doctors will harvest herbs and sometimes kill animals to extract certain essential substances from their bodies; this is all violence. Āyurvedic texts recommend that doctors perform certain rituals and ceremonies to mitigate the results of this violence. Of course, such doctors will also receive positive karma at the same time because of their good deeds, but these should be considered separately. As we have discussed, good deeds do not automatically offset bad deeds. A doctor must still address the effects of his having caused pain.

In some cases we may need to act in self-defense to protect ourselves from other people's violent actions toward us. In such cases, it is our duty to shield ourselves from serious harm so that we can achieve Realization in this lifetime.

CULTIVATING NONVIOLENCE

Many wonderful benefits result from nonviolence. Those established in ahimsā solve many problems within the family, the society, and the nation. The best way to cultivate nonviolence is to have a close connection with a yogi who follows the principles of nonviolence. In his presence all forms of animosity will diminish. There are two varieties of animosity. One is temporary; it lasts for a certain amount of time and then disappears. The other type is by birth. This is the inherent hostility that a mongoose has for the cobra, a cat for a mouse, or a lion for a deer. In the presence of one who is established in nonviolence, both types of enmity will be dissolved. There are many accounts of animals that have this sort of instinctual animosity toward one another living peacefully together in the presence of one established in nonviolence. Human beings are affected in the same way in the presence of such a yogi. Just being in the presence of a yogi trains and shapes us in such a way that even after we leave the yogi, we maintain the principles of nonviolence. The next best thing is to cultivate friendship with those who honor nonviolence. This will develop a shield from violence in general.

If we cannot be in the presence of one established in nonviolence, then we can cultivate empathy and compassion. We need to develop the skill of projecting ourselves into the skin of another. We need to understand that her Soul is the same as ours. If, through violence she is feeling pain, then we can feel that same pain. We develop this ability by gradually developing love for each and every thing in this universe.

SATYA: TRUTHFULNESS

The second yama is *satya,* or *truthfulness.* Satya relates primarily to our gift of speech and how we use our words. Humankind has been given speech through the grace of Nature. Though birds and animals also have the ability to express themselves, it is a far more developed capability in humans. As the crown of Nature, human beings have the unique capacity to experience the physical, divine, and spiritual spheres. As such, we have a greater capacity for knowledge and emotions, and we experience this universe in meaningful ways. Our mind has the capacity to function like a very powerful lens; it can observe the most minute, subtle, and hidden details of this universe. It is through our words that we are then able to communicate these treasures of experience and knowledge to others.

Our words can also be used as a tool, an ornament, a weapon, or a shield. Humans have been granted the freedom to behave as they like. But this freedom is conditional insofar as one reaps the results of one's actions. Speech can be used for the welfare of one's self and others, or it can be used for ruin. In this way, one must hold a tremendous amount of responsibility in regard to one's words. Through words alone, one can carry an individual to experience divine bliss or great suffering.

However, as the grace of Nature, speech is designed to communicate the truth. The very purpose of truthful speaking is to support the welfare of all beings. But this should be done carefully. Knowing the power inherent in speech, our first responsibility is that it should not harm at any cost. We should understand that a truth told at the wrong time, in the wrong place, to the wrong person, or in the wrong situation, is either told in vain, or may cause irreparable damage. This is considered a grave misuse of our words and a deep misunderstanding of truth.

TRUTH AND THE ETERNAL TRUTH

Our tongues are meant to speak truthfully in ways that inspire interest in others about the Eternal Truth. Truthful speech facilitates the experience of the Eternal Truth and the bliss that accompanies it for all humankind. The Eternal Truth shares certain characteristics with other forms of truth, but few are able to speak about it directly. Even a yogi cannot explain it fully, because the experience of the Eternal Truth is beyond words. However, if one is able to express this experience even partially, he can enlighten others and encourage them to experience that same Truth. Even if one cannot fully explain that final experience, one may aim to at least stir longing in others to desire the possibility.

Each human being has a right to live with the knowledge that the Eternal Truth is at the heart of the universe, and that it is possible to have a direct personal experience of it. Speech is meant for explaining the disciplines that eliminate the imbalances and impurities from our lives that prevent us from realizing the Self. The more we hear about yogic disciplines, the more we are inspired to move toward the yogic condition. When others encounter teachings about the existence of the Eternal Truth and the proper use of this external world, they will be motivated to keep their lives in balance. Gradually, they will begin practicing on a yogic path.

ONE'S LIVELIHOOD AND TRUTH

Each human being needs to earn a decent, honorable livelihood. Sometimes that requires us to do mundane work and to talk about many things not directly related to the Eternal Truth. An accountant must talk about money and taxes. A physics teacher must communicate with his students about the laws of the physical universe. An automobile mechanic must talk about pistons and spark plugs. But, if we always keep the goal of Realization in mind, and if we are earning a decent livelihood so that we can maintain our body to reach that goal, then talking about accounts, physics, or spark plugs is also considered meaningful.

Regarding the external universe, there are many lesser truths that we can speak of with confidence. If these lesser truths are linked with the Eternal Truth, then they are considered to be true. If by his words, a teacher is able to fan the spark of divine aspirations in a student's heart, then what he says is true. Or if these truths support our path toward the ultimate, they are considered to be true. When we are honorably taking care of business in this external world, attending to our duties with the intention of supporting our path toward Realization, what we say is considered to be true.

While discussing anything in the universe, aspirants must be reflective before speaking. Their introspection and observation will offer them knowledge that is available from no other source. If they are asked a question, their deep contemplation will link them to the truth.

This connection, however subtle, will lead them to speak truthfully and greatly facilitate their progress on the yogic path.

There is another remarkable benefit of steadfast honesty. Once one is *fully* established in truthfulness, a reliable link is established between the truth and one's words. From that point on, whenever one's word energy is manifested in the external world, it will be associated only with the truth. Nature uses such a person as a device to propagate truth. Whatever she declares will be true, and many truths will emerge even without her knowledge. Her system will operate as a conduit to bring forth the Truth. This is a wonderful benefit to the entire world.

At the height of such achievement, this person will have the power to bless or curse. Whatever she pronounces shall come to pass. This achievement will operate in two ways, one even more wondrous than the next. First, her internal capacity will increase and expand, and she will become an immensely powerful person. Second, she will become an agent of Nature, carrying blessings and curses to others. This is certainly the grace of God, because when there is some error in the universe, such a person can bring the correction though a blessing or curse. Furthermore, the beneficial results of good and honorable actions will also manifest immediately. In the presence of such a yogi, karmic resolution need not wait for the next birth. Such a person deserves to be honored alongside the deities.

WHEN TRUTH CAUSES MORE HARM

All yamas are not equal in importance. Patañjali listed nonviolence first because nonviolence is of the highest priority. The paths of both nonviolence and truthfulness must be followed strictly. However, where truthfulness is in conflict with nonviolence, preference will be given to nonviolence. The yogic definition of truthfulness maintains that we should speak the truth only when it does not harm anyone else. If anyone's welfare is undermined, then even if we are saying something "true," it is not considered to be truth in the ultimate sense of the word. Though something may be objectively true, it may end up causing harm to both the speaker and the listener. For instance, if speaking a truth interferes with someone's path to the Eternal Truth, it will result in karmic repercussions for the speaker. Thus, both will suffer.

There once was an āśrama where some students were studying with a Realized teacher. One day a deer came running out of the woods and into the compound. The sage and his students all watched with amazement as the frightened creature ran into the cowshed. They were exclaiming about this when a hunter, armed with bow and arrow, came into the āśrama. It was obvious to all that he was in eager pursuit of the deer.

He approached the sage and his students asking, "Sir, did a deer run past here?" The sage answered, "Yes, it did." Eagerly, the hunter asked, "Which direction did it go?" The sage pointed vaguely and said, "It ran away." The hunter quickly ran past the cowshed and out of the hermitage in the direction the sage had pointed.

One of the students felt disappointed and shocked that his teacher would lie. He began to wonder what other misleading deeds the sage might be capable of. The sage understood the student's feelings due to his yogic sight. However, he kept quiet. In his wisdom, he decided to wait for the appropriate time to impart the required lesson.

The next day, the sage decided to visit another āśrama some distance away. As he would often take a student or two with him on such a journey, he asked the troubled student to accompany him.

At some distance from the āśrama, while walking along a deserted section of road, they were suddenly accosted by a group of *Kāpālikas*. These Kāpālikas were members of a violent cult who worshiped a deity to whom humans were sacrificed. Once a year, they would go in search of an offering to their goddess. Though they would not choose women or children, they would seek a suitable male offering for their ritual. They would bring him back, sacrifice him, and bury him in their sacrificial grounds. As fate would have it, the Kāpālikas were hunting for such an offering on this day.

The Kāpālikas overpowered the sage and his student. Quickly, and without mercy, they bound the two with tight ropes. After the travelers were immobilized, their captors placed them on horses and proceeded to the sacrificial grounds.

Though his usual nature was to be brave and ambitious, the student was terrified to the core of his being. He began to sob. He remembered his parents and friends, fearing that he would never see them again. He began to mourn these last moments of life, and he had deep regrets that he was about to die so young. In contrast, his teacher remained silent and calm. His face betrayed no emotion.

After some time, the sobbing student noticed the quiet state of his teacher. Though he was too upset to think much about it, he was surprised and found it strange.

The unlikely captives were transported to the sacrificial grounds, where they were greeted with shocking enthusiasm by an entire tribe of Kāpālikas. The sacrifice was to be performed before dawn the next morning. The sage and student were tossed into separate tents nearby to await their fate. Exhausted from hours of grieving, the student fell silent and began contemplating his terrible luck. As he quietly began to accept his fate, he developed a plan.

At dawn, the Kāpālikas came to take them to be sacrificed. The student made a request to speak to the leader of the cult. The leader came and stood impatiently before the student, demanding he speak quickly. The student began humbly, "Sir, first of all, I will tell you that I am quite ready and willing for you to sacrifice our lives to your great deity." This startled the leader. No one had ever said such a thing before, and he was suddenly curious to hear what the student would say next.

The student continued, "You are doing a noble deed, and certainly pleasing this deity, by your obedience and devotion. I have come to understand what a wonderful honor it is for me, and this old man to be sacrificed to your deity. But an offering to this great deity should be pure and perfect; otherwise, this goddess will be greatly dissatisfied. Alas, honesty forces me to disclose some unfortunate news to you before you proceed. The two of us are not perfect, nor pure. I, for one, was bitten by a dog and have a festering wound on my leg." The student feigned difficulty walking, greatly exaggerating what had been a small wound he had received the previous week. Then he continued, "But even more seriously, as you have no doubt noticed, my companion has had no reaction to being captured by your men. This is because he is deaf, mute, and mentally deficient. He doesn't understand that he is about to be sacrificed. Surely, no man in his right mind, knowing what is about to happen to us at this moment, would stay calm and quiet!" Gathering courage, he concluded, "Please consider this all very carefully. We are ready to go and be sacrificed, but you should take care that your sacrifice is worthy."

The leader turned to the members of his group. They whispered among themselves as they imagined the wrath of their insulted deity. They reexamined their prisoners and came to a hurried conclusion that what the student had said was true. They finally decided it best to release the sage and his student.

As soon as the two had traveled a good ways away from their captors, the student stopped and bowed down before the sage. With great emotion he conceded, "Sir, please forgive me for mistaking you. I now understand the relationship between truthfulness and nonviolence. I intentionally told those lies back in that camp, because, had I not done so, we would now be dead. As we waited for dawn, I recognized how tragic it would be if you were to lose your life before your virtuous work in this world is complete, and I were to lose my life before Realization. You have shown me that life is very precious and must never be wasted. Certainly, lying is a dishonorable act, but *the sin of telling these lies is small when compared to the tragedy of our deaths.*"

Through his yogic sight, the sage actually knew ahead of time how the events would unfold. Even before being caught by the Kāpālikas, he knew exactly what would happen, down to the last detail of their escape. His intention to subject himself and his student to such an experience was to teach the student about the value of Realization, and the precedence of nonviolence over truthfulness. Because human life offers the possibility of Realization and the potential for happiness, it is precious beyond measure. When we value truthfulness above the preservation of life, or the goal of Realization, we act in ignorance.

TRUTHFULNESS AND KARMA

The story of the sage and the student offers an extreme example. But this same principle is true even in less critical situations. If someone has an opportunity to realize the Self, we must avoid hurting his chances of doing so. Any truth that we tell must not disturb one's progress toward that goal.

If at all possible, we must try to avoid difficult situations where there will be some pressure to say something that might hurt someone.

However, if we do find ourselves in such a situation, we need to consider which path will incur the mildest repercussions. We must choose the lesser of two evils.

When we commit an error, karma is the result. This karma drives our actions in life and creates repercussions that we must experience, either in this life or the next. We create karma when we lie. We also create karma when we destroy life or allow it to be destroyed. The second category engenders far greater consequences than the first. On the other hand, if a yoga practitioner tells a lie to avoid destruction of life, she may feel confident that she has done her duty. Certainly, telling a lie is a wrong action, and the practitioner will need to seek forgiveness or experience some corrective action. But it has much less impact than taking life or allowing a life to be taken.

Let us say a man with a severe heart condition consults a doctor for a frank assessment of his condition. He urges the doctor to tell him the exact truth about his disease. A good doctor will be able to determine whether the patient is capable of receiving such information. If the patient is not able to receive the truth, the doctor will play down the seriousness of the disease and instill a hopeful attitude in the patient. He might cushion the impact of his prognosis by saying, "Yes, there is a problem, but it can be managed with some changes in your diet and a little exercise." He might offer the patient some medicine as a simple "precautionary measure." However, if the doctor thinks that the patient is likely to expire within the week, and if he recognizes that the patient could really not bear to hear the direct truth, the doctor will withhold that information. In this situation, if the doctor told the truth, it would be a form of violence. There are cases in which doctors have shared the full truth with a patient, only to have the patient die soon thereafter because they could not withstand the shock.

As in the Hippocratic Oath, a doctor's first duty is to "Do no harm." The first priority for a practitioner of Aṣṭāṅga Yoga is to practice nonviolence and to preserve life. Subsidiary to that is to tell the truth. On a deeper level, truth is *not* actually subordinate because the very purpose of truthfulness is the welfare and happiness of humankind. Truth should enlighten us in such a way that happiness results. If by telling the truth we cannot help someone, it is better to remain silent.

Alternatively, we must find a way to tell the truth that causes the least amount of harm.

TRUTH IS THE ETERNAL TRUTH

Full truthfulness, like total nonviolence, is not possible 100 percent of the time. At its deepest and most profound level, truth *is* the Eternal Truth. It is what yogis visualize during the yogic experience. The only thing that is absolute, fixed, certain, and unchangeable is the Eternal Truth. The only way to tell the ultimate truth is to talk about the Eternal Truth. That alone constitutes unmitigated truthfulness. However, there is a paradox: While visualizing the Eternal Truth, we are unable to talk, and while we are talking, we cannot visualize the Eternal Truth. Again, this is because mind ceases to function in its customary manner.

RELATIVE TRUTH

What remains beyond the yogic experience is the physical world, which represents relative truth. Since everything about this external world changes constantly, how is it possible to tell the truth about it? This dilemma is further exacerbated every time someone asks us a question. There is a particular context to every question, but we may not always fully understand what that is. For instance, in Mysore, India, there is a large hill overlooking the city called Chamundi. On top of that hill, there is a very beautiful, old temple with the same name. Someone might ask, "Have you seen Chamundi?" We might answer, "Of course, I have seen it! How could I miss it?" However, this questioner might be referring to the temple alone, and not the hill! Such ambiguity is one reason the sages advocate that we should talk less.

If we have been acquainted with someone for many years and someone else asks whether we know that person, we might say we know the person very well. But this is not really true, because we only know a very small aspect of each person. Given the ever changing nature of the universe, even the aspect we knew yesterday is altered in some way today. There are many similar kinds of "untruths" that occur in everyday life. Everyone accepts this. Yet, in practicing truthfulness, it is best to avoid even these minor infractions. The more we talk, the more we invite the opportunity to tell a half-truth, or even a lie.

Teachers sometimes use the following demonstration to illustrate this principle. They place a pot in front of a student and ask whether he can see the pot. The student answers, "Yes, of course. It's directly in front of me!" Then the teacher points out that the student sees only one side of the pot, and only from one angle. There might be a big crack or hole in the pot on the other side, or it might be painted with a different design or shaped in a different way. And if the student were to look inside of the pot, he could not see the outside and vice versa. Our vision gives only a partial picture. Such are the limitations of the five senses. Therefore, it is often very hard to tell the exact truth about anything. Most of what we say represents only partial truths. Given that this is unavoidable, we are left with the same advice: Talk less.

The Buddha taught various discourses to his students. Four of these students listened to his teachings and developed four different paths. Someone went to the Buddha and asked him why four different paths were developed from the same teaching. He replied that it was because of the individual and unique nature of the saṃskāra the students brought to their understanding of his discourses. Each disciple would give extra emphasis to some aspects of the teaching while neglecting others. In this way, the Buddha's disciples unintentionally twisted and altered the teachings because they were unable to hear them precisely without their own bias. It was not possible for them to repeat the truth as the Buddha originally explained it. When a Realized person is describing something, the listener may unknowingly twist the information as it is being received. How then can we say that it is the truth?

LIMITS TO EXPRESSING THE TRUTH

To visualize the Eternal Truth, a yogi must go into Samādhi. Then, after emerging from Samādhi, he must attempt to impart some aspects of his experience, even though he will then already be far away from it. That is why the Eternal Truth is considered as *anirvācya,* a term that means "it cannot be explained." A yogi cannot carry the totality of that experience to the world. However, he can carry a part of it, and it is his duty to do so.

During the night, we may have a wonderful dream, but after we awaken, we can recollect it only partially. Much of it will be forgotten. When we sleep, our mind goes partially inside. But it does not go to the very depths, the way it does in the yogic experience. The difficulty in talking about a dream is small compared to the difficulty in talking about Samādhi. After experiencing that condition, yogis are unable to describe it in depth. When they try, the words will not convey their experience. Hence, they cannot speak the ultimate Truth. However, it is possible for sages and yogis who have experienced it to speak of it to some extent. Even that may lead others to the same experience.

Sages of the past would acknowledge when they did not know something about a particular subject. That is part of their greatness. If someone asked a yogi about something he did not know, he would promptly say, "Oh, I don't know anything about that." When we talk about anything in the universe, we should give information only to the extent we know. If we do not understand something, we should say so in a straightforward manner. If we are teaching something to others, we should always set the proper expectation in their mind. We should be frank in our teaching and acknowledge, "I know something, and I'll teach you what I know. Beyond that, you need to seek elsewhere." We should not mislead anyone. This is an important aspect of satya.

When a student is cultivating an intention to become Liberated, he will naturally honor truthfulness. If he lives with a yogi who is established in truthfulness, he will be able to understand its value fully. As a result, he will begin to develop satya as his practice. Gradually, this practice will grow. He will talk less, so that there is less chance of lying. He will take much care over every word and sentence that he utters, developing a deep consciousness of truthfulness. Whenever there is a chance of lying, due to karma, he will think about the adverse impact it will have on his life. He will listen more keenly, thus inviting in the Eternal Truth to influence his words when he does speak. Gradually, the tendency toward truthfulness will gain strength, and over time, he will establish himself in satya.

ASTEYA: NONSTEALING

The third yama is *asteya,* or *nonstealing.*

If we look around us, we see objects everywhere. Which of these really belong to us? Do we have a right to own these things? Which objects do we really need for our use? Which should we leave for others to use?

We may borrow some tools or other materials from our neighbor. An honorable man will treat such tools with even greater respect than his own. Good parents teach their children to always return borrowed items in the same condition or better. In the same way, all objects and various forms of materials belong to Nature. As the children of Nature, we are allowed to use them, but only temporarily. It is as though we have a wealthy friend who trusts us implicitly. If we honor and respect that friend, we will not abuse the trust she has placed in us. We will use only what has been loaned to us specifically. If we have been refused certain materials, and they have been loaned to somebody else, we will understand that that is the prerogative of the owner.

Nature allows us to use material objects for limited periods of time. When we desire some food, it is best to cook and eat it immediately, or it goes bad. When we buy an automobile, it gradually breaks down as we drive it, and we sell it or give it away. Even a house, which appears to be permanent, also deteriorates, albeit more slowly. Even our closest possession, our body, withers with age. When we purchase a house or some land, we use it for a while, but inevitably we move on. Even if we stay in the same house until we die, we eventually leave it and all of our possessions. We even leave our body. Nature gives us the clear message that we do not really own anything, and the materials we hoard are only loaned to us.

When we adopt the view that everything belongs to Nature, we become restrained in our use of material objects. We carefully consider whether we really need to use a particular material. How much of it should we use? Are we using it for the right purpose? Is it useful for us or for someone else? Will it be harmful if we use this material, because Nature intended it for some other use? If we have this wider view, our tendency will be to choose materials carefully. This is the first principle to be understood in the practice of asteya, nonstealing.

Misunderstanding this principle leads to an incorrect sense of ownership. If we do not properly honor this principle, we will inevitably engage in various forms of stealing, knowingly or unknowingly. To eliminate such problems, yogis recommend that as we use and acquire materials, we remember to whom they belong. In addition, they recommend that we use these materials only to please God. Then there will be no question of stealing.

Though all materials belong to Nature, we are still allowed to own them for various intended purposes. The *intention* we have to own a particular material is partially what develops our attachment to it. If this material is then stolen, the intention stays with it. As a result, the mind and body of whomever steals it from us will be disturbed. It also disturbs whoever uses or claims the stolen material, knowingly or unknowingly. This is one kind of negative influence that results from stealing.

Stealing develops negative karma that is carried into a person's next birth, where it will result in some corrective action. Even more significantly, stealing develops a saṃskāra that will recreate the same tendency for stealing in subsequent births, thus leading to repeated cycles of pain and suffering.

Let us try to further understand the influences that result from stealing in the example of the following story.

There was once an honorable monk who was fully disciplined in his practice. His mind was quiet and controlled, and his body was pure. He had a cloth, a staff, and a bowl to carry water. These were his sole material possessions. As part of his discipline of detachment, he never stayed in one place for more than one night. Each day he would travel to a different village. Sometimes he would stay in someone's house as a guest; sometimes he would sleep on the steps of a temple.

One day, a Brahmin invited the monk for a meal at his home. The monk readily accepted. When the Brahmin went home and asked his wife to prepare the midday meal, the two discovered that they did not have enough food in the house to feed their guest. The Brahmin honored the monk and wanted to show proper hospitality, so he left his house to look for food. As he passed his neighbor's garden, he saw a beautiful assortment of fully ripened vegetables. He reasoned to himself that it would not be a problem to take the vegetables since he was offering them to such an honored monk. He also thought that, were he to ask his neighbor, the neighbor would surely give permission. So he gathered enough of the vegetables for a fine meal. He brought them home, and his wife prepared various delicious dishes and served them to their guest. The monk enjoyed the meal and found it fully satisfying.

Afterward, the monk and the Brahmin were sitting at leisure on the front stoop of the house. The Brahmin had a cow grazing nearby with her new calf. This particular cow was very beautiful, delicate, and of a golden color, which is considered auspicious. She was very gentle, and her calf was healthy and bright. The cow and her calf stopped their grazing and meandered to their cowshed behind the Brahmin's house.

The monk was oddly taken by this cow and calf, thinking they were exceptionally beautiful animals. He suddenly asked the Brahmin to give them to him as an offering. He imagined how he might travel with them and how they would provide him with milk, ghee, and other precious products.

Somewhat surprised by the monk's bold request, the Brahmin replied that the cow provided the main sustenance for his life. He could not manage without her. He apologized and explained that he could not bear to part with them. The monk, however, could not give up the idea of owning this cow and her calf; he became obsessed with the idea. The next day, the Brahmin was called to go to another part of the village. The monk seized this opportunity to steal the cow and calf and then left the Brahmin's house.

As he was walking to the next village, the monk suddenly felt astonished by his actions. Never before in his entire life had he stolen anything. Moreover, being so fully disciplined, he had few if any cravings for material things. For many years, he wanted nothing more than his cloth, stick, and bowl. He quickly repented for his actions and decided to return the animals and ask the Brahmin for forgiveness.

When he arrived at the Brahmin's house, the monk approached him and explained what he had done, begging for forgiveness. Being a kind and generous man, the Brahmin easily forgave him.

After the animals had been safely returned, the monk pondered deeply. How could this have happened? Why had he suddenly stolen something for the first time in his life? He knew that he did not have the nature of a thief. It was all exceedingly strange. He began to ask the

Brahmin a few questions: Was the Brahmin earning his money in an honorable way? The Brahmin replied that he was. How had the Brahmin acquired this cow and calf, his house, and the other materials on his property? The Brahmin explained how each item had come to him in an honorable way. Then the monk asked how the Brahmin had acquired the food he had served to the monk. The Brahmin explained how and why he had taken the vegetables from the neighbor's garden.

The monk suddenly realized that eating stolen food had been the source of his thoughts and desire to steal the cow and calf. He explained to the Brahmin how the food had been made impure because it was not purchased or gathered in an honest fashion. The Brahmin understood and repented for his wrongdoing. He promised he would not repeat such a deed again and asked for the monk's forgiveness.

If the stolen food had such an impact on the monk who was maintaining such rigorous disciplines, how much greater would the impact be on a common man? The monk was able to identify the misguided thought in his mind and eventually link it to the impure food that had caused the imbalance. Most would not be able to make this kind of association so easily and would end up performing unwanted actions without ever knowing why.

OWNERSHIP

The ownership of materials affects our lives in many ways. Ownership has the capacity to disturb our mind when meditating, thus causing changes to or modifications of the mind. Although all materials belong to Nature, we tend to think that they belong to us. A man will look at the watch on his wrist and think, "This watch is mine." In this way, his mind is attached to the watch. When someone declares to himself that a certain material belongs to him, this declaration has a tangible impact on the material. A yogi with a clear and objective mind can easily sense this influence on a material.

True ownership of any material is illusory. A material we have now was not originally in our possession, nor will it be at some point in the future. Though we will have it only temporarily, we *feel* that we will own this material forever. This is a delusion on our part, though our attachment may be extremely strong and very real.

As we saw with the monk who ate the Brahmin's dinner, if an article is stolen, the theft's influence will be carried with it, and the one who uses the stolen material will feel the influence. Further, the original owner of the material feels pain when losing it. That pain is carried through the material and affects the thief. He may not recognize it, but it will be there. If by chance we receive some stolen material, it will create vṛttis, or modifications of the mind, for us. These vṛttis have an effect on all facets of our life, especially on our meditation practice. Even if that material changes hands many times, the mind's influence will be carried along with it.

There is a story about a Westerner who was hiking in the Himalayas. High up in the mountains there is a sacred spot, a cave, where exists a stalagmite in the shape of a *Śiva lingam,* a large cylindrical-shaped stone representing the power of Lord Śiva. Many Hindus go on a *pravāsa,* a holy journey, in order to witness it. Near the end of the journey, there is only a footpath, because the mountain is too steep and rugged for a road. The Westerner was one of many making this pilgrimage. One day, after resting alongside the path, he accidentally left his shoulder bag with all his valuables sitting in open view. He proceeded on his way for several hours. Upon discovering his loss, he quickly retraced his steps. To his great surprise, he found his bag in the same spot he had left it. Even though hundreds of pilgrims had passed it, the bag had not been moved an inch. None of the spiritual seekers who noticed the bag would touch it, because it did not belong to them. They all knew the spiritual purpose of their journey would be denigrated if they were in possession of something that belonged to someone else.

We need to have this same discipline in our lives. If something is not ours, we should not even touch it if possible. Or, if appropriate, we may take it to a lost-and-found. But if no such place is available, then we should let it remain.

A Realized yogi may likely possess a few materials, whether simply for his work or survival. Because his mind is unconditioned, he will be unattached to the material, and he will not think of himself as its "owner." He may, however, have an intention to use the material for a particular purpose, such as the welfare of humankind. Even though the yogi does not have a possessive mentality, the effect of his mind on the material will be strong. If someone were to steal that material, it would disturb the thief tremendously.

The influence and power of the mind are far greater than we might imagine. One day my Eternal Teacher, Śrī Raṅga, went with his closest disciple to purchase some bananas at a shop. In any given bunch of bananas, some will be smaller, and some will be larger. The disciple selected one particular set of large bananas. Śrī Raṅga immediately said, "No, better to select a different bunch." Though the disciple did not understand, he obeyed and chose different bananas. He then paid for them, and the two of them left the shop.

Once they were alone, the disciple asked, "Why did you not want that first set of bananas? They were beautiful, large, and perfectly ripe."

Śrī Raṅga replied, "The first bunch of bananas was desired by somebody else. It had a bad influence. You can go ask the shopkeeper about it."

The disciple returned to the shop to inquire. The shopkeeper told him that only a few minutes before my teacher and his disciple had arrived, someone else had come to the shop and wanted that first set of bananas. But that person had thought the shopkeeper's price was too high. He had left the shop, criticizing the shopkeeper.

This customer's mind left an influence on the bananas. This influence lasted, even though he had left the shop. A common man could not see this effect of the customer's mind on the bananas, nor was the disciple able to discern it. However, the yogi could detect its subtle effects because of the high capacity of his mind.

There are three types of stealing. The first is theft, which everyone is familiar with. The second is plagiarism, and the third is mental stealing. These latter two can be even more significant than the first.

PLAGIARISM

A knowledgeable teacher is an abundant treasure of information. If by his grace, he teaches us something, we should not impart that information to others without his permission. He taught us with a specific purpose in mind, and we need to use the resulting knowledge for that purpose only. It is his asset, and he has shared it with us through his mercy. If we use the knowledge improperly, or without his permission, Nature considers that to be plagiarism, or stealing of words.

Even if we have permission to teach this knowledge to others, it is our duty to acknowledge our source. When we acknowledge our source, we link ourselves more closely to it. When we are closely linked, we will continue to receive knowledge from that source. Thus, we encourage the flow of truth in our direction and may maintain the right to share this truth with others.

When we fully acknowledge our source of information, the receiver will also become linked to the source and not to us. Otherwise, we do a great disservice. Our mind contains less knowledge and information than that of a Realized yogi. After giving what we know, our reservoir of information will be drained. Those whom we are teaching will soon become disillusioned. By fully acknowledging our source, we can encourage others to go to the original teacher once our own level of understanding has been exhausted.

MENTAL STEALING

There are many different kinds of confidentiality we must honor and respect if we want to become established in asteya. Many times someone will ask us to hold some piece of information in confidence. This must be fully honored. In the same way, we should never read someone's personal diary, letter, or document without permission. To do otherwise is stealing. Even overhearing another's words is a form of stealing. If possible, we should shield ourselves in some way or even move away from the conversation if possible. If we cannot avoid hearing something, we should hold it in confidence and repeat it to no one.

In the great Indian classic the Mahābhārata, there is an important figure named Droṇācārya. Not only was he a yogic personality, he was also a wonderful instructor in the arts of war and archery. Archery, in those times, was different than it is today. Arrows were considered to be more than mere physical weapons; they were infused with the energy of mantras. When they were shot from a bow with precise intention, the arrow would follow the victim until it pierced him. Using another mantra, the arrow would spread fire, burning everything in its path. With a third mantra, the arrow would generate a huge wind, strong enough to destroy the enemy. Droṇācārya was an expert in this type of archery. He was a master of mantras and the practice of making arrows sacred. He would infuse an arrow with a particular energy from his own body and send it off to do its work.

At one point, Droṇācārya traveled across the country in search of some suitable students. One day, he came upon a group of royal princes. (These young men would later become the principal characters in the *Mahābhārata.*) The princes had been playing with a ball that had accidentally fallen into a deep well. The well was narrow without any steps. The princes were gathered around the well looking at their ball far below in the water and wondering how they were going to retrieve it.

Droṇācārya asked them why they were all looking into the well. The princes explained about their lost ball and pointed to it at the bottom of the well. Feeling compassion for the young boys, he picked up a blade of grass, infused it with the energy of a sacred mantra, and threw it into the well. To the astonishment of the princes, the blade of grass dropped to the bottom of the well and returned with the ball!

The princes thought this was marvelous. Filled with admiration and awe, they returned to their father, the king, and explained what Droṇācārya had done. The king quickly assessed that Droṇācārya was no ordinary man and sent for him. Droṇācārya came and introduced himself. He admitted that he was knowledgeable about archery and the art of warfare. So the king begged Droṇācārya to take up the task of educating his sons. Thus, Droṇācārya accepted the honorable position as the preceptor of the princes.

One of the princes was Arjuna, who would later ride in battle with Kṛṣṇa as his charioteer. Arjuna was a noble, holy boy of divine birth. He had extraordinary capacities. Droṇācārya took an oath that he would make this beloved student, Arjuna, the best warrior in the universe.

One day, a hunter's boy, named Ekalavya, came from a nearby village to the palace where Droṇācārya was teaching the princes. This boy had a passionate intention to learn archery. Ekalavya asked Droṇācārya to be his teacher. However, Droṇācārya was fully engaged with teaching the princes. It was his holy obligation to reserve himself for the princes, so he told Ekalavya, "No, I regret that I cannot teach you. It is my duty to instruct these princes. Please search somewhere else for your education." Ekalavya was terribly disappointed with this response. Nevertheless, he saluted Droṇācārya and bid farewell—though he was not ready to release his desire to be taught by this great master.

As Ekalavya traveled home, he carried Droṇācārya in his heart. He believed Droṇācārya to be the best archery teacher in the world, and that if he were going to learn archery, he must learn from this teacher. Because of his extreme interest, honor, and love, the image of Droṇācārya was burned into his mind. Unbeknownst to either Droṇācārya or Ekalavya, the teacher had been initiated into the student's heart.

Ekalavya returned to his home and made a statue of his hero out of clay. It was an extremely accurate statue, capturing every minute detail of the master's features, so that it conveyed the very essence of Droṇācārya. He placed the statue in a highly honored place, where he meditated upon it regularly and began practicing archery. Because of his meditation upon the image, a transmission gradually took place. Ekalavya quickly gained much of Droṇācārya's knowledge of archery.

By chance one day, Droṇācārya and the princes were out hunting with a prized hunting dog near Ekalavya's village. The dog would run in front of the hunters, seeking out prey. When he discovered some animal, he would bark to signal the hunting party. At one point, the dog detected the presence of some animals and started barking loudly.

Ekalavya happened to be practicing his archery with full concentration and found the noise disturbing. Even though he could not see the dog, he shot seven arrows through the forest, using only the sound of the dog's barking as his target. He shot these arrows with such skill and precision that they did not kill the dog, or even wound him, but simply entered the dog's mouth and closed it so he could no longer bark. The bewildered dog ran back to his owners.

Upon seeing this dog and the arrows sealing his mouth shut, Droṇācārya and the princes were amazed. It was obvious this was no easy feat; rather, it was a high-level achievement. They directed the dog to search for the archer who had done this and soon found Ekalavya practicing his archery.

Droṇācārya did not recognize Ekalavya but noticed the lifelike statue of himself. Immediately upon seeing Droṇācārya, Ekalavya fell to his feet to honor him. Droṇācārya demanded, "Who are you, and what are you doing?"

Ekalavya replied, "I am your disciple. If you will remember, I came to you for instruction, but you refused me. Since I considered you to be the best teacher for me, I started practicing archery here in my village, making a statue of you as my teacher."

Droṇācārya questioned the boy further to find out the extent of skill he had gained. He was astonished. Nearly all the knowledge in his mind had been transmitted to Ekalavya. The boy knew many, many wonderful techniques and mantras that Droṇācārya had not even taught to Arjuna, his best student.

At first, Droṇācārya was simply struck with wonder at Ekalavya's knowledge. However, upon reflection, he felt dismayed. He had taken a solemn oath to use his knowledge for the welfare of the princes only. This included teaching Arjuna to become the best warrior in the universe. Moreover, Droṇācārya's knowledge was enormously powerful; if placed in the wrong hands, it could have terrible consequences for the kingdom itself. Because Ekalavya had taken his knowledge without his consent, Droṇācārya was forced to acknowledge that an unwitting, but nonetheless serious theft had occurred. To right this wrong, something more than acknowledgment was needed.

Years ago in India, teachers were not paid while the student was learning. Instead, at the end of the student's education, as a duty, the student would inquire if there were anything the teacher specifically required. This was considered a gurudakṣiṇā. Sometimes the teacher would stipulate, "There is something I need to further my intention to bring knowledge to the world. Find this and offer it." The student would never refuse his teacher's request.

So, after thoughtful consideration, Droṇācārya told the boy to give him a gurudakṣiṇā. The boy quickly said, "Yes, master, I will give you whatever you like." Droṇācārya replied, "Please offer your right thumb." Without hesitation, Ekalavya cut off his thumb and offered it with sincere contrition. Not having a thumb to grasp the bowstring hindered his practice of archery forever.

While this may seem like an extreme example, it clearly demonstrates the principle of mental stealing. As with other forms of stealing, it leads to unforeseen consequences and disturbances for others. It is harmful and not a fitting method to gain knowledge.

CARRYING A LASTING IMPRESSION

If we have ever stolen anything, we likely still carry an impression of that misdeed. But there are steps we can take to eliminate it. The first step is to fully repent and to take a vow that we will never again touch materials that belong to somebody else. Then the best thing to do is to give the stolen item back to the same person and request his or her forgiveness for our wrongdoing. We must attempt to make the victim feel as though the theft had never happened. However, sometimes this is not possible. That person may have died, or we may not even know who they are. In such a case, we need to perform some form of penance and offer the same or similar items to a person in need. This reduces, or may even eliminate, the negative karma formed by the theft.

ELIMINATING A TENDENCY

To eliminate a tendency to steal, we are best served by practicing charity. Generosity will solve many of the imbalances that create the desire to steal. First and foremost, it develops nonattachment to materials. Rectifying the problems of stealing may take some time, but continued generosity over a long period is one of the prerequisites.

According to Patañjali, if one feels the temptation to steal, he should contemplate the many negative impacts of his stealing. This alone, in due course, will eliminate such tendencies.

Even while eating a handful of food, it is our duty to ask permission from Nature. This may be done as a small prayer, or simple acknowledgment. Nature is like our Mother, and it is our duty to ask and thank her for what she offers us.

Patañjali tells us that when someone becomes established in asteya, she will naturally experience abundance, receiving wealth and the best materials in each and every category: the best cow, gem, land, house, and so on. This is actually a kind of yogic *siddhi*, or power. One well established in asteya will naturally attract all the best materials in her lifetime. This is not to suggest that only honest people will enjoy prosperity. There are many cases of dishonest individuals accumulating vast wealth while others suffer in great poverty. Much of this can only be understood by assessing the individuals' karma and saṃskāra. Without the hindrance of negative karma or saṃskāra, those established in asteya will experience its fruits.

This is a law of nature. Human beings are the crown of nature because they alone can experience the ultimate happiness of the Eternal Truth. Properly used materials are very meaningful to all of humankind. They provide enjoyment of bhoga and support an aspirant on the yogic path. Stealing materials is like trying to wear another's clothes. They do not fit properly or serve our body's needs. In fact, their energy will lead to many disturbances throughout our entire system. If non-stealing is firmly established, and our systems are properly maintained, we will attract many precious materials in this world. In return, these materials, in their own purity and preciousness, will benefit our overall welfare. These are some of the reasons we must firmly cultivate asteya in our yogic practice.

BRAHMACARYA: MOVING TOWARD THE ETERNAL TRUTH

One evening, a man was walking down a street when he recognized a close friend standing under a streetlight looking for something on the ground. He said, "Hello, my friend. What are you looking for?"

"I have lost my car keys," his friend replied.

Naturally, the man joined in the hunt. After ten minutes, the man and his friend had closely examined the entire area under the pool of light. The man declared to his friend, "I am sure the keys are not here. Tell me exactly where you were standing when you lost them."

Suddenly looking up, the friend answered, "Oh, I was about fifty yards down the road."

Exasperated, the man exclaimed, "Well, then why are we looking under this streetlight?"

His friend replied, "The light is better here."

This is our problem. We look for our happiness in a place where it does not exist. But first we need to uncover the fundamental desire in our mind. What are we searching for? Why are we collecting, possessing, and using so many materials? What drives such an insatiable appetite for happiness?

We need to go within and stop searching for this happiness externally. We need to return to the point where it was lost, which is at the heart of our being. Instead of trying to flush it out of endless layers of worldly affairs, we can follow a method of experiencing intense joy directly. We can follow practices and disciplines that move us toward the Eternal Truth. This requires some education about the mind: How do we quiet the mind? And what will happen when we do? As we learn about our yogic path, we will begin to practice new techniques that help us accomplish these goals. At the same time, it is essential that we adopt a way of life that supports us to move in this direction. When we do this, we are practicing a form of brahmacarya.

In Saṃskṛta, *Brahma* is "Eternal Truth," and *carya* means "movement." *Brahmacarya* literally means "moving toward the Eternal Truth." This is the fourth yama we will discuss. Sometimes brahmacarya is incorrectly translated as control of sexuality, or celibacy. While it has a relationship to celibacy, it is not the same. True brahmacarya is the discipline of keeping the body and mind attuned for Realization.

Everyone wants happiness, but most are ignorant about the true nature of happiness. A greedy man striving for riches is really searching for happiness. A musician with a one-pointed focus on becoming famous is no different. A person who spends several hours a day exercising and grooming his body believes that those activities are the key to that elusive state. Many people believe that if they can find the right mate, all their dreams of "happily ever after" will come true. There are myriad ways that we search for happiness. We desire one type of happiness but chase after another.

We believe the happiness we seek is to be found in the material world, but what we truly want is the happiness of the Eternal Truth. Every desire is actually driven by the underlying yearning for Realization of Brahma. Our desires are ways that we actually crave the Eternal Truth. We are simply unaware of it.

Realization of the Eternal Truth brings a state of bliss that is essential to every aspect of our being. Everyone works hard to find it, but most are looking in the wrong places. In this sense, every human being is a *brahmacāri*—but this is an *indirect* form of brahmacarya and will not yield the same results as a more direct form of practice.

There are two varieties of direct brahmacarya, based on the constitution and saṃskāra of the aspirant. The first variety is followed by a householder with a family and everyday responsibilities who also practices for Realization of Brahma as an integral part of his lifestyle. The second variety is for the intense practitioner who is fully immersed in his practices, ideally without the responsibilities of family, job, and so on. There are two types of these intense practitioners. The first is a *youth* who dedicates himself to this kind of intense practice but only until he marries, after which he will live as a householder. The second type is the *monk* who vows to practice intensely throughout his entire life.

SEXUALITY

Various cycles of energy in our body affect us at particular times throughout the day. One wakes us up at the same time each morning; another causes us to have an appetite at certain times throughout the day. Sometime around midday, we feel energy that supports us to focus on our work or job. In the evening, we are more relaxed and sociable. At roughly the same time each night, we begin to feel sleepy and have a strong desire to go to bed. Likewise, if we pay close attention, we will recognize that at sunrise and sunset, our system offers the greatest support for meditation practice.

A person with a supportive lifestyle can do various activities throughout the day and develop harmony with the body's natural rhythms and cycles. Besides balancing things like our digestive system, sleep cycle, and capacity to do productive and meaningful work, such a lifestyle will fully support a person's ability to meditate. This is the most important reason for developing such awareness.

Like many of the other rhythms in the body, there will also be a cycle for sex in each individual. Sexuality is the grace of Nature. The primary purpose of sex is to produce a child whose qualities are equal to, or better than, those of the parents. For this, certain disciplines are required. The parents need to be compatible, and they need to have full commitment to each other and toward maintaining a supportive way of life. *Both* must have the intention for Realization. With these disciplines in place, sex becomes infinitely more meaningful. Such a lifestyle, including sex, is the practice of brahmacarya.

Traditionally, however, people would not refer to such a person as a brahmacāri. That title was reserved for intense practitioners: young boys who had not yet sexually matured or married. An intense practitioner will devote himself singularly and totally to yogic practices. He will also abstain from sex. This is how the title of brahmacarya became equated with celibacy.

Sex is an innate desire. There are āśramas where hundreds of men are celibate. Though they forcibly control sexual contact, they compensate with many other material desires. Consequently, their minds are not necessarily moving inward toward the Eternal Truth. They are dwelling in the external world rather than in the internal world. Even though they are celibate, these people are not brahmacāris.

Rarely, a few individuals will have little or no attachment tendencies, including any sexual desires. This is something different from impotency. When a common man is impotent, he may still have a desire for sex, he simply will not be able to engage in the act. Someone who is fully detached from sex, as well as from other material desires, is a rarity. Monkhood is recommended *only* for this type of individual. To force a lifestyle of monkhood is not recommended in yogic disciplines or advocated in an ideal way of life.

STAGES OF LIFE

Each person passes through many different stages in life. If one is living an ideal lifestyle, sexual desire occurs only during particular stages in one's life. If there are no unnatural external influences, this period typically starts around the age of sixteen and continues until the age of eighty. Males and females will differ somewhat due to a female's more prominent physiological and biological role in bearing children. Her monthly cycle will be a constant reminder of this. However, serious concentration on the internal path delays the onset of sexual maturity. In that event, it will not commence until the age of twenty-four to thirty-two, or possibly as late as age forty-eight, in extreme cases. Prior to this, a practitioner naturally does not think about sex. In part, this is because he is fully immersed in realizing Brahma or one or more of the sacred arts and sciences.

Many other factors also contribute to his detachment from sex. With the proper education and understanding he will have the patience and understanding to wait until he is married. Also, many types of nonvegetarian foods stimulate sexual urges, as well as foods like onion, garlic, and eggs. Such a practitioner will not consume these foods or visit places that stimulate inappropriate sexual interest.

The only desire an intense practitioner, referred to as a *naiṣṭhika brahmacāri,* will have is for realizing Brahma itself. Because of this serious intention, he will always be involved in his practice. He will meditate for many hours each day. At other times, he may read books or engage in other activities in full support of his practice. This practice is primarily recommended for men, because a woman's body will experience a monthly downward flow of energy connected to her menstruation cycle. This cycle must be highly honored. For a woman, the practices of a naiṣṭhika brahmacārya would contradict her body's natural flow of energy.

YOUTH

Society today has become relatively incompatible with a yogic way of life. In traditional yogic society, boys and girls were not permitted to socialize with each other very often. On occasion, they would meet at family gatherings, where they would regard members of the opposite sex as brothers and sisters. This practice helped to preserve their purity and capacity for meaningful growth and development. When boys and girls are placed too often in close proximity to each other, they are free to look at each other, talk to each other, and have physical contact. Even though this may seem benign on the surface, or even deemed by many as healthy, it fosters early sexual maturity.

This idea may seem strange to one who lives in a Western society, where liberalism is the prominent ideal. Unless we think about this issue within the context of Realization and Liberation, it can be challenging and difficult to understand. When the primary goal of an *entire* society is Realization, a social convention such as limiting free association between the sexes makes practical sense. If young people are allowed to practice yoga in an ideal setting, they may attain Realization early. When a youth attains this spiritual state as a teenager, she can greatly benefit society and the world. Moreover, she will enjoy her entire life to an unimaginable extent.

Sexual maturity is not bad. It is necessary for a content and happy household. However, early sexual maturity is an enormous detriment to early yogic achievements. The two are incompatible. It may seem like a trivial issue, but when it prevents or hinders the path toward Realization, it is a catastrophe.

SEXUAL EDUCATION

It is best to avoid teaching a young child about sex. It will provoke untimely sexual maturity. All information needs to be taught at the appropriate time, so that it will not disturb the child's psychology. When we plant a seed, we need to provide fertilizer that is appropriate for a newly sprouted seed. Later, when the tree is fully grown, we need to supply a different type of supplement that will help the tree to produce fruit. Childhood is meant for education, to understand certain aspects of the universe and the Self. We need to allow that process to proceed uninterrupted. When the child reaches an appropriate age, and when we see signs of sexual maturity, we may provide some information about sex. We need not teach everything about sex directly. Some of the information will be taught by nature; the rest is our duty to teach with sensitivity and awareness.

The mind of a very young child will be pure like a clean slate. If a child between the ages of five and eight commences yogic practices such as devotional chanting, sitting calmly and quietly, and learning about Realization, he will easily develop an inner awareness and a capacity to sense his inherent connection to the Divine. Children, by their nature and innocence, stand at the door between the internal and external worlds. Rather than encouraging children to be extroverted, we should provide food for their heart, to feed their inward natures. The process for their development will take its normal course, providing the environment is conducive to practice. After brahmacarya is practiced for a number of years, sexual maturity will arrive naturally. When it does, it is time to marry.

If an adolescent is sexually provoked, his desire must be artificially controlled and suppressed, because there is no outlet for it. This can have adverse effects on the youth, including the onset of emotional and mental disturbances. Therefore, if one is ready for sex, he should also be ready for marriage. If he is not prepared for marriage, he should have some counseling from a person who can speak to him with compassion and understanding to help explain the dangers of his untimely interest in sex.

EDUCATION AND GENDER

In an ideal society, brahmacarya means that the practitioner will follow many disciplines. One such discipline limits contact with the other gender. In India years ago, even brothers and sisters would refrain from sitting together or touching each other after the age of eight. Instead of spending a great deal of time in each other's presence, all were encouraged to be fully involved in their own education, particularly about the Eternal Truth.

At an early age, boys began attending special schools, or *gurukulas*, and āśramas. When they were fully absorbed in their education, brahmacarya occurred naturally in their bodies and minds. It was not a matter of restricting or suppressing their sexual instinct. In light of the strong focus of their life, they did not think about the opposite sex.

In the past, the traditional Indian approach for educating females was to educate them in their own homes. Their father, uncle, or some other suitable elderly person provided their spiritual education. It was important that their teacher be aged, so there was no possibility of any sexual provocation.

While these ideals were once suitable for Indian culture, today much of this cannot be implemented, even in Indian society, because modernization is so prevalent. It is a difficult problem. Most families have no choice. They must send their children to school, and most schools practice coeducation. If they do not send their children to school, the children may become isolated and not learn how to relate adequately to other children. Nevertheless, it is important to remember some of the traditional practices in educating children. Perhaps in the future, a society will emerge where they can be followed.

Even today, however, we can find same-sex schools. Often, the motivation for them is for children to learn better by studying with other students of their own gender. The reason is that they are less likely to be distracted by the opposite sex. While this is certainly an advantage, it is a lesser consideration when compared to its impact on the child's yogic path.

We must bear in mind that only one hundred years ago, many of these ideals were implemented in societies throughout the world. Historically speaking, the idea of coeducation is a new one. Even in the Western world, most schools were not coeducational. These days, it is not considered sophisticated or modern to espouse the idea of gender separation in schools. Rather than making a decision based on what is popular, we need to carefully consider what is truly most valuable. Will a decision yield a desirable or an undesirable effect? What impact will it have on the individual's ideal growth?

The ultimate goal for all human beings is the same, regardless of where they live. Although people in other countries need not rigidly follow the same practices as seen in traditional India, meaningful lessons can be gleaned from close observation of these practices. Regardless of social structure, or individual differences of constitution, all societies struggle with similar challenges in today's world. Enormous problems have arisen from children being overexposed to sexuality in media, schools, and other social structures. This is why it is so important to develop a basic understanding of what best supports an ideal yogic way of life, then choose for yourself what works with your life.

SEXUAL PROVOCATION

Sexual provocation is of two types. One type derives from society at large. It is not possible to drive through a city or surf the Internet without seeing provocative images in advertisements and elsewhere. The other type of sexual provocation comes through our own interest. If we find ourselves constantly interested in sex, then we are provoking ourselves and further developing this interest. We cannot control the provocation that society instigates, although we can decide to ignore it. But we can control the provocation that stems from within. We can totally eliminate it if we choose. It is a practice, and like other practices, it requires a level of self-discipline. For example, after marriage, couples must stick to their vow to have sexual connections only with one another. If someone else entices them, they can refuse the invitation. This practice alone would be a solid step in the direction of developing an ideal society.

There are other things that an aspiring brahmacāri can do. Those who are not married and want to follow the principles of brahmacarya need to avoid sexual activity completely. Later, if they wish, they can marry. However, the marriage should be totally committed, and the couple should teach yogic ideals to their children.

Another practice of brahmacarya is to avoid unnecessary physical contact. In general, it is best not to be too casual about physical contact with other people. In our effort to maintain balance and clarity within our systems, we should avoid taking on the influence of other people's physical energy. However, we need not be too radical in our solutions. These days it is difficult to live without touching. Hugging is a common practice in the West. In moments of extreme love, compassion, and mercy, neither party is likely to be injured by a hug because of the beneficial energy flow between two people's systems. Aside from these situations, however, if people frequently and mechanically hug, it has the potential to cause energy clashes. These may be recognized or unrecognized. Here, too, we should at least note that such contact was not seen one hundred years ago. Even in the Western world, it was rare for unmarried men and women to share a casual embrace. And kissing was tantamount to an engagement for marriage!

IN SUPPORT OF LIBERATION

Within a marriage, sex has the capacity to support Realization. This is for two reasons. First, the supreme pleasure enjoyed in sex can support meditation. It can help build a person's capacity for the supreme joy that he or she may then experience in Samādhi. Second, the proper use of sperm and ovum may bring a new life to the world. This child may achieve Liberation, especially if both the father and mother intend for the child to Realize the Self. If both parents understand some basic principles and disciplines about how to conceive and raise a child, the child may easily achieve Realization and Liberation. If a member of any family achieves Liberation, all that person's relatives will be greatly supported to achieve Liberation, as well. Therefore, if such a spiritual child takes birth, the parents will progress in their path with less effort, as well. In that case, having a child fully supports brahmacarya.

RESPONSIBILITY AND COMPATIBILITY

Sometimes a female feels the need for sex while her husband may not be interested at that particular point in time. The yogic principles of brahmacarya advise that he should satisfy her needs. Her body and mind have a need to feel the touch and closeness of her husband. If he does not provide this, she might develop thoughts of being with someone else. This would disturb both the husband and wife, and, further, it would disturb their children. If her husband does not satisfy her, he has neglected his duty. His behavior would be out of alignment with the disciplines of brahmacarya. The disturbance of one-sided sexual interest will be rare when both the husband and wife practice certain disciplines.

In the same way, the female has the responsibility of meeting her husband's sexual needs. If the male has sexual desire and she does not fulfill it, he may think of another woman. If either the husband or wife does not understand this aspect of brahmacarya correctly, he or she is in danger of destroying the balance in the entire family. To maintain the disciplines of brahmacarya properly, teachings need to be imparted directly or indirectly to both men and women about the significance of sex and its meaningful use.

NATURE'S DISCIPLINES

Animals will follow precise cycles for sexual activity. As a rule, they will initiate sex only during the months when provoked by Nature. We do not normally see such patterns for human beings, however. The main reason for this is that most human beings are not living according to certain natural principles and disciplines. Due to the characteristics in their constitution, animals have no choice but to live in accordance with nature. They go to sleep and wake up by nature's clock. They eat whatever is provided—they never prepare foods and keep them in the refrigerator. All aspects of an animal's life align with Nature's principles.

Naturally, sexual desire will increase in the spring and lag in the summer. Many animals have sex in yearly cyclical patterns. We can see some aspects of this pattern in human beings; it is Nature's influence. However, human beings have developed modern conveniences that artificially alter many aspects of a more natural way of life. Additionally, many people are in the habit of artificially provoking sexual desire as a way to try to find happiness. For these reasons, we see sexual desire at inappropriate times of the day. However, if both the husband and wife follow some basic yogic disciplines, their sexual desire will gradually become more synchronized. There may be a variance of a few hours, but the cycles of husband and wife will be nearly identical. As a result of their committed love, radical changes will take place over time that can smooth over any differences in cycles, and they will maintain compatibility with each other.

CONCEPTION

Human sexuality is evolved from the natural instinct to bear a child. Many Souls are waiting to get a human birth. In this way, it is also our duty to have children. But our aim should be to have a noble child. This is a great responsibility for the mother and father.

If a couple wants to have a child who has noble qualities, they must observe a few disciplines. First, they should attempt to live as close to an ideal way of life as possible. They should develop a very serious intention to bring a noble child into the world. This establishes a *saṅkalpa*, a powerful intention toward this specific outcome. This saṅkalpa will play one of the most significant roles in conceiving a noble child.

The time of day that conception occurs has a tremendous influence on what Soul takes birth. Just as sunrise and sunset are sattvic periods in the day, which support the mind to move inward, and midday supports our jobs, there is a specific time that is favorable for sex and conception. This is normally during the night, a little past midnight.

Hence, there is an optimal time of day to both enjoy sex and conceive a noble child.

Ill-timed sexual activity deeply disturbs harmony in the system and may lead to undesirable qualities in a child. It disturbs various mechanisms in the body and mind, creating emotional imbalances. We should avoid sex at sunrise, sunset, and midday. Unfortunately, it is a broad and much more complex subject than we can address in this book. However, if we accept some of the basic principles, and physically and psychologically prepare for that instant of conception, then our system will automatically support the outcome we desire. If we are in harmony with these principles, and observe a few disciplines, sexual enjoyment and conception itself can be an integral part of brahmacarya.

MARRIAGE

Many factors must be favorable to bring a child into the world. A couple needs to have a suitable means of livelihood to support a family. They need to have an adequate living space. If these favorable conditions do not exist, it is not wise to have a child. For example, if they are in college, they need to be devoted to their education. However, a natural sexual connection will still provide joy and relaxation. In doing that, it supports the couple's yogic practice. Yoga never professes that sex is wrong. It only suggests that sex be enjoyed according to Nature's principles.

There are a few basic disciplines for married couples to practice. It is best to refrain from sexual contact in the daytime, at sunrise, or sunset. Daytime is for work, and sunrise and sunset are for meditation. In addition, there are a few precious days each year, marked by the Indian lunar calendar, that are particularly beneficial for meditation. One such example is *Mahā Śivārātri,* which celebrates Lord Śiva. Sunrise, sunset, and precious days are meant for introverted activity, and sex is an extroverted activity. To have sex at those times is an inappropriate use of energy. Yogic philosophy warns that if we conceive a child at those times, the child may be unfit for meditation. It will have many counterproductive qualities. Yogis have verified this many times in India. Sincere yogic practitioners will readily abide by this principle.

The ramifications can be serious for the whole family and can bring grief throughout the entire life of a child conceived in the wrong way. Needless to say, it greatly hinders yogic practice.

In addition, yogic tradition maintains that the man and woman are best served to sleep in separate beds. There are several reasons for this. One is because sleeping in the same bed artificially provokes sexual desire. Another reason is that both husband and wife will simply enjoy a more peaceful sleep. If one partner moves, it will not disturb the other. Also, their energy will not influence each other. The night hours are meant for deep rejuvenating sleep; we should minimize any disturbance to this. It is one of the most important prerequisites for a healthy life.

NATURAL RHYTHMS AND CYCLES

There are many different activities and duties that we must attend to in our lives. These include food preparation, meditation, and work. We can artificially stimulate our systems to perform these duties and activities at any time. It is no great challenge to artificially provoke hunger. If we are constantly looking at food, smelling it, and tasting it, we might eat eight meals per day, but it would not be healthy to do so. Similarly, it is far better to avoid provoking sexual desire at unsuitable hours. Sexual desire will arise at the right time automatically, like our hunger, if we live according to Nature's principles. Periodically, it tells us, I am here. Please attend to me. We need not eliminate it, but rather we should attend to it at the right time.

FREEDOM AND SEXUALITY

There is a lingering attitude in the West that advocates the liberty to do whatever we want, whenever we want to do it. This includes the freedom to have sex with no restrictions. This is evident in the common practice of having sex before marriage. This same kind of thinking maintains that any limitation on sex amounts to repression and close-mindedness. Let us inquire into what constitutes freedom and what constitutes repression or bondage.

In this physical universe, those beings that lack an understanding of their original condition and purpose are held in bondage by their suffering and attachment. The most meaningful definition of *freedom* is release from that kind of bondage. For this, we need to implement right thought and a right way of life. Then, like the young prince in the beginning of this book, we will gradually remember who we are, where we came from, and where our original kingdom lies. Finally, we will attain Liberation, the real freedom. Until that time, we must undergo various forms of suffering. All will experience this dilemma; some will recognize it for what it is, and some will not.

For example, sometimes out of necessity, a man will need to work hard for years. Every day, he must labor to the maximum extent possible in order to meet his obligations. Perhaps he has a big family to support. When, by chance, such a man gets some free time, he may not know what to do with it. He might feel that he is being idle and wasting his time. This free time may feel like a burden, even a kind of bondage. This man has become so accustomed to his obligations, they no longer feel oppressive; rather, freedom itself feels oppressive.

This is the nature of our mind. We develop attachment and affection for what we are used to, whatever that may be. We form attachments to our friends and associates, no matter who they are. We might seem to enjoy our lives with or without disciplines. We feel comfortable living in compromised situations, and improved alternatives may even look unattractive to us.

A person might enjoy sex very much and feel that this is an expression of his freedom. However, the idea that freedom involves undisciplined sexual activity is a misconception. This person has forgotten what true freedom is. Given the possibility of Liberation, such "free sex" is the opposite of freedom. It actually increases one's bondage because of the unintended disturbances it causes in each individual. It is an act that has an enormous impact on the mind and body. Actions that carry that much impact should be done with great care and awareness.

It appears rare in the West for one to abstain from sex before marriage. However, there are ways one can reduce the impact of previous sexual experiences on one's practice. First, one should make a new commitment to have sex only after marriage. Then allow previous sexual experiences to be part of the past. One should not fantasize about them nor hold on to any pain they may have caused. These experiences should simply be put out of one's mind to minimize their impact.

The most basic principle of brahmacarya is to enjoy one's life to the maximum extent through Realization and Liberation. This is possible only when one maintains a certain discipline around sexuality. Sexuality is not condemned; it is even recommended. The proper use of sex brings much happiness, and it can support our path to Liberation. As with many other forms of enjoyment, if one's sexuality is developed upon certain yogic principles, it will enhance one's overall welfare and lead one to Brahma—Eternal Truth.

APARIGRAHA: DETACHMENT FROM POSSESSIONS

Aparigraha is the fifth yama, and it teaches us the value of having fewer possessions. Often explained as "nonhoarding," aparigraha encourages us to only possess what is most necessary and to reduce our tendency to accumulate too many belongings. The practice requires us to become keenly aware of various materials' negative influences. Ultimately, aparigraha helps us develop nonattachment. In the Yoga Sūtras, Patañjali suggests that *abhyāsa,* or practice, and *vairāgya,* or detachment, are the two most important prerequisites to attain Samādhi. In this way, it supports us on our path toward Liberation. Through the practice of nonattachment we free ourselves from the hindrances and negative influences that are associated with materials.

Long ago, there was no need to amass excess material possessions. Most needs could be met by what nature readily provided. This was partly because there were fewer human beings, and their needs were simple. Each person collected only what was needed. There was little reason for collecting and storing extra possessions.

As the population gradually increased, demand grew, and materials became increasingly scarce. Simultaneously, a tendency toward greed and a habit of accumulation developed. These tendencies have been slowly evolving over the past few thousand years, undergoing a tremendous surge within the past few hundred years, and greatly influencing our present day.

LESS IS MORE

As we have made clear, there is no harm in enjoying material things in our world. The problems arise when we begin to crave and acquire them in excess. Whatever we acquire with ease should be received with gratitude and enjoyed to the fullest. On the other hand, those things that are not important, and require great effort on our part to acquire, we should forget.

For instance, there are hundreds of varieties of food, but in order to be healthy and fit for Realization, we need to eat only a few of them. Once we establish a basic diet, we may or may not decide to eat other kinds of food. We are best served to work hard only for what is most needed to maintain a balanced mind and body. This is our duty and the essence of aparigraha.

We actually require only a few possessions in this world. If we develop contentment with what we have, it is easy to avoid accumulating more. We will think, for example, "This handbag is old, and it is no longer in fashion, but the strap is strong and the compartments are the right size. It suits me just fine." Perhaps our kitchen appliances are no longer new and shiny, but if we are able to use them to cook nutritious and delicious meals, we will be content. The overall result will be that we are happier. This is aparigraha.

BE CAREFUL ABOUT WHAT YOU ACCEPT

A major facet of the practice of aparigraha is to be able to distinguish what is appropriate to possess, and what is not. Someone may have an abundance of a particular resource and offer it freely to us. Even though it is free, we should still ask ourselves, "Is it beneficial to receive this or not?" If it is essential, we can accept it—no problem. But if it is being offered with an expectation of something in return—be it money or something else—we might reconsider. When there is an expectation, we need to fulfill that expectation. Otherwise, the object will affect us adversely. A friend or acquaintance may offer a meal to us in her home expecting that on some other occasion we will offer a meal to her in our home. This is actually a type of business transaction. We may decide to accept the offer, but we have to complete the exchange.

If objects are not useful to us, we should refuse them. Let them go somewhere else where they will be useful. The intention behind this principle of aparigraha is to avoid a kind of enslavement to material objects, and to reduce their unwanted influences. If we closely examine our lives, there is really little need to have many materials. Most often, we can live happily without them.

Overconsumption of materials is a waste of our life force. Ownership also implies responsibility. Most of our possessions require some form of maintenance and upkeep. It is our duty to care for what is in our possession. This takes time and precious energy. For example, we must simultaneously earn enough money to buy goods and to buy a house to store them. In the West, I have discovered the phenomenon of people even renting storage units, simply to store materials they may never use again! This kind of behavior can easily lead to unwanted stress in our lives and prevent us from fully tending to our yoga practice.

Yoga points to a more sane approach that benefits us and the world at large. It is far better to depend only on those materials that are most essential to our lives and our ultimate goal in life. When we aim to purchase a new item, we should ask ourselves, "Is this item useful directly or indirectly for my well-being? Does this material support a yogic lifestyle?" The truth is that human beings actually require few materials. We require a simple and adequate house for shelter. We require two or three simple, tasty, and nutritious meals each day. We require a few articles of clothing. And we should allow a few articles for pleasure and sheer enjoyment. That is essentially all we need.

HOW OUR POSSESSIONS INFLUENCE US

We have already mentioned that material objects have an effect on every aspect of our life, including meditation. Their influence is of two types. The first is external, entering and influencing our system via our five senses. The second is internal. Each object is made up of energy and therefore has a life of its own. This energy affects our system internally. We must ascertain whether we want that material's influence. Will that energy have a beneficial or harmful impact on our life and yogic practice? If the impact of the energy is harmful or unknown, and we really do not need that material, why would we take the risk? Whether we are aware of it or not, a material's adverse effects may far outweigh its seeming benefit.

The universe has a purpose for each material and object. All of these materials are made up of energy, and this energy wants to flow in alignment with its purpose. Purchasing some object and bringing it to our home can often be like building a fence around this energy. If the material is not meant for us, it may cause an unwanted impact on different aspects of our lives.

There is a round, black stone one can find in the Gandiki River in Nepal. This stone is known as *saligram*. It is considered a very precious material, because it acts as a medium for various divine energies. Indians honor the saligram and regularly worship it. Ancient Indian texts describe the many different effects these energies may have on a person or family when the stones are brought into a home. They warn that it is important to select the right stone, so as not to bring an unwanted, disturbing energy into the home. Today, many people collect these stones, unaware of their potentially disturbing effects.

We live in a world today where objects come from distant places and have been manufactured in all sorts of ways. We are rarely aware of the people who labored to make these things, or under what conditions they worked. Nor are we aware of the negative impact these items may have had on the environment. Many of these objects may carry negative influences that it would be best to avoid having in our homes.

Objects influence our mind through our emotions. They can provoke a wide range of emotional states. These may range from anger to peace and contentment. Some may bring sadness, others joy, and still others jealousy or egotism. At times these influences are naturally inherent in a material. At other times, the material carries the influence of its previous owner. This is why, as previously mentioned, stolen objects are disturbing to their current owners. Even a beautiful or sacred sculpture or painting may cause adverse influences if it has been stolen. This is also why it is not advisable to collect old items in the home, like antiques and other previously owned objects. Despite our intentions, we may never be sure of the exact history of these items. It may be impossible to know who their previous owners were, or whether they may even have been stolen and resold at some point.

Based on previous births, a person may have the karma and fate to have many materials. In such a case, this person may receive materials through an inheritance. She does not need to reject this. Rather, she may enjoy these things to the fullest extent, so long as she does not crave them or collect them unnecessarily. Perhaps in that previous birth, she desired something but was unfit to possess it because of some other karma that was at work. In this current birth she may now be fit to possess such a thing. If she does not get attached to it, she can enjoy it without any negative repercussions. This will not hinder her yogic practice. The important question to remember is "How attached am I to this material?"

WHEN IT IS GOOD TO ACQUIRE MORE

Sometimes because of certain situations, it is inevitable to collect or even amass a few items. At the time of harvest, a farmer will possess a vast quantity of food. Since he may not receive much food until the next harvest, it is his duty to store enough to last until that time. Nature gives the food only at the time of harvest; this is Nature's indication that it is acceptable to store some food until the next harvest.

In the same way, if we live in a climate that has cold and hot weather, this requires two types of clothing. However, we need not purchase new warm clothes every year. At the end of the cold season, we can simply store the warm clothes until the following year. Storing some materials, so as to avoid unwanted and excess effort in the future, will not disturb our life; rather, it can actually help simplify it.

Years ago, families were often closer. Parents could rely on their children to provide for them in their old age. These days, family life is more complicated. There may be no feasible way for the children to provide adequately for their elderly parents. Given this trend, it is often necessary to save some money for retirement. We should not have to live in poverty during our old age, but we also need to think carefully about how much we will require and aim to accumulate only that amount. We should be careful not to let fear of the unknown drive us to panic and feel we never have enough.

It is wise to give serious thought to all decisions about accumulating possessions. We need to carefully consider whether we are proceeding in accordance with Nature's principles or artificially manipulating the situation. Sometimes this is difficult to determine. We need to look deeply into each of our actions and decide if our need is genuine or based on confused thinking. Over time, we will come to understand what is required and what is not.

MIND AS SKILLFUL MAGICIAN

Many people collect material objects to make them feel good and secure. What they really crave is the happiness that comes from the Eternal Truth, but they do not know how to find it. When an individual acquires a material object that satisfies a craving, the mind's activity is reduced for a short time. That person will have fewer desires temporarily because they have satisfied one desire. The mind has a great capacity to play tricks on itself, but even tricks of this most skillful magician can be unveiled if we pay close attention. The material is never the cause of happiness. The source of such happiness is a quieting of the mind's vibrations, not the object itself. Until we understand this, we will be bound to endless cycles of temporary pleasure followed by renewed craving for some new material. Instead, we must look within our own heart, to the source of true happiness.

There is another problem that keeps us attached to the material world. It is ignorance. We think material possessions lead to enjoyment, but actually they lead to more problems. Sadly, we tend to ignore the problems and focus only on the small enjoyment they bring. The root of this misconception is our hasty thinking, which short-circuits the mind's capacity to see what is really happening. As a result, we cannot accurately measure how much we have actually enjoyed these materials, or how many problems they have created for us. This is how we mistake our misery for happiness.

ATTACHING OURSELVES TO THE ETERNAL TRUTH

When the proper goal of life is not set, we automatically become attached to the things of this world. There is a direct method to reduce our attachment to these materials. The solution is to establish our life's purpose with firmness and determination. After we have done this, we will come to recognize how counterproductive it is to attach ourselves to materials and objects that are irrelevant to our primary goal. Detachment comes about naturally when our primary goal is properly set.

The mind is like an inchworm. Unless the front of the inchworm is attached, it will not release its back end. If we want to become detached from material objects that do not bring happiness, we must attach ourselves to the source of true happiness.

But how can we attach ourselves to the Eternal Truth? We can do so either directly or indirectly. The direct method begins when we receive some education about the goal of Realization. This can lead us to begin a yoga practice to help quiet our mind. This will provide encouragement and validation as to the existence of the Eternal Truth. If we clearly focus on Realization of the Eternal Truth, the objects of the external world will lose their importance. This is the *direct* method.

Sometimes it is not so easy to set our goal properly. We continue to struggle with many questions. What is human life? How can it best be used? What is happiness? Why are we craving possessions? What is the role of these possessions in human life? Is there a way to be happy without so many possessions? The spiritual education we receive is most important. Superficial teachings will not support us. The teaching needs to be from heart to heart, from one who fully understands the source of happiness. A skillful teacher will impart useful information to a student. The student is in need of that knowledge; otherwise, he will continue to struggle with attachment tendencies. If a Realized teacher properly conveys the answers to all these questions, the student's attachment tendencies will completely stop.

The *indirect* method is to attach ourselves to such a teacher. This establishes an indirect attachment to Liberation. As we become more and more attached to the teacher, everything else will automatically become less important. We will look around us and objectively see that many things and many activities in this external world are not important. We will easily become detached from all this activity. This is the indirect method.

A PATH OF LEAST RESISTANCE

Yogis say that we do not need to worry about our attachment tendencies. We have an innate tendency to be attached, and it is not possible to force detachment. Instead, we should become adept at deciding where to attach ourselves. We need not even understand all the ways that we are attached to the external world. It is very difficult to study all of our attachments and know their source. Sometimes the source is saṃskāra from previous births. In this case, by the influence of māyā, our mind is unskilled in understanding the nature of our attachment. Consequently, the sages tell us to deemphasize our focus on our attachments. Instead, we need to set our target properly; then our attachments will naturally relax and release. This is the simplest method of detachment.

A university student who has a deep interest in her studies will forget many other affairs. In contrast, a student who is very interested in cricket or baseball will forget about her studies. She will develop a kind of detachment from her lessons. This is the nature of the mind. Yogis tell us to set our goal; the rest will occur naturally. At some point, we will become detached.

TOO MUCH INFORMATION

The practice of aparigraha not only applies to material possessions, these principles can also be used to understand the effects of acquiring too much information.

There are two ways that we can avoid acquiring unnecessary information. First, we can simply avoid listening to gossip. Sometimes, if there is an argument in our neighbor's house, we will be very eager to hear the details about that clash. But such information will not help us toward our greater goal in life. Another example involves the Internet. Some people spend an enormous amount of time engaged in reading and listening to unnecessary information. While social media sites serve humankind in various beneficial ways, they can also deliver gossip from all over the world. For the most part, it is best to limit our exposure and even ignore these kinds of unnecessary information. Too much information dries the heart and steals happiness.

Second, it is prudent to avoid unnecessary intellectual information. There are many fields of study in the external world, including physics, natural and theoretical sciences, mathematics, and engineering. Music, literature, dance, and spiritual drama are subjects associated with the spiritual world. While measured study in any one or two of these areas can be beneficial, it is impossible, and undesirable, to study all these things. This is not meant to discourage learning. Rather, this is intended to encourage the use of discrimination in deciding what to study. This is too is aparigraha.

A GOAL TO SEE CLEARLY

Ownership of many possessions is more disturbing than beneficial to our lives. If some of those objects are not meant for us, we will lose our peace of mind by using them. When disturbed, our mind is not capable of clearly seeing this life, let alone past lives. In the Yoga Sūtras, Patañjali explains that one who is established in aparigraha will come to understand his previous births.

If we tread lightly in this world, using only those objects that we truly need, our mind will be at peace. We can see more about ourselves. We can even understand aspects of our previous births. This clarity will help guide us on our yogic path to make the right decisions and act accordingly. If we do not strive for such clarity, we will be bound to endless cycles of temporary pleasures, followed by renewed cravings for more. Our goal instead should be to simplify our lives so that we may more easily experience what we truly crave: the Great Light and true happiness that we possess within ourselves.

DAYĀ: MERCY

The sixth yama, *dayā,* or mercy, builds our capacity to express our compassion for others. If we are firmly established in dayā, and we see a woman who is physically ill or in pain, we will be moved to alleviate her suffering. We may offer her support to see a doctor, or suggest a simple remedy that we can provide. Perhaps we can take care of some other worry for her, run an errand, or offer some food so that she can concentrate fully on her recovery. Or we might be able to offer some kind words that will relax her mind. Sometimes a person simply needs someone to listen to him as a way to sort out his problems. These are all ways of showing mercy toward others.

A FORM OF GRACE

Self-Realization and Liberation require grace. We have a large capacity to bestow Nature's grace on others. Showing mercy is one way Nature uses us to bestow grace on others. We can support others with our thoughts, our physical strength, or our material possessions. We can use whatever strength or capacity we have for the welfare of others. When we show grace toward others, we pave the way for grace to flow toward ourselves.

As we develop a capacity to show mercy, our body will gradually become a conduit for the flow of Divine Grace. When our body becomes a medium for grace, more divine energy will flow in our system. Not only will it benefit others, it will benefit us, as well. Showing grace to others welcomes it into our own lives. Showing mercy toward a sick person indirectly paves the way for removing sickness in our own lives. If we show mercy toward someone who has any type of problem, it helps alleviate our own problems.

Why is this? To answer that question, we must first understand why we have problems. We have problems primarily because of our negative karma. We have done something inappropriate in the past, and problems arise as repercussions of those actions. This karma will show us the errors in our behavior and lifestyle, and we must suffer the consequences. For example, if we insult a teacher in this life, we may be reborn a teacher in our next life—in order to experience the pain of such an insult ourselves.

If we show a lack of repentance for our misdeeds, it will be difficult to correct the tendencies in our behavior, which lead to such errors in the first place. The consequences of our wrongful actions will expand until we fully comprehend we have made a mistake. We will be caught in a vicious karmic cycle.

When a criminal in prison sees the error of his ways, and the authorities see that the criminal fully understands where he went wrong, they will sometimes reduce the prison sentence. Similarly, when we have a serious level of repentance in our system, our suffering will be reduced. This is a law of Nature. The very purpose of karma is to bring correction to our system.

Showing mercy to others shows our comprehension of the laws of cause and consequence. It helps us to develop a natural tendency toward repentance. Showing mercy engenders repulsion toward wrongdoing. This will gradually dissolve much of our karma and greatly support our yogic practice.

Dayā will be the yogic path for some. They show full mercy toward each and every person. It is a practice that is rooted in love and developing an open heart. This is all that is necessary for them to practice. When taken to its fullest extent, dayā will solve most of their problems. When their problems are solved, Self-Realization will come easily and require no further effort.

ĀRJAVA: STRAIGHTFORWARDNESS

The seventh yama, *ārjava,* means "straightforwardness." If an aspirant maintains the strict practice of straightforwardness, gradually his system will exude a wonderful flow of energy from within. This is because there are no obstacles to hinder the natural flow of this energy. When we hide something, we establish a block, so that others will not understand our real intentions. If we dam a stream, not only do we block the water, but we block the fish, as well. Ārjava eliminates our tendency to create screens or blinders in our mind; it develops a capacity to easily receive right knowledge, and it lessens strain in our system.

We have three main tools to use in this life. The first is our mind. The second is our words. The third is our body. For these three to work together optimally, there needs to be harmony and consistency between them. There must be an alignment between our words and our thoughts, our actions and our words, and our thoughts and our actions. Using these three tools, we are able to perform many virtuous works in this world, as well as cause a great deal of trouble. Ārjava helps to establish an open flow of energy and easy collaboration between these three essential tools.

NATURE'S EASE AND DIRECTNESS

We see straightforwardness almost everywhere in nature. For the most part, animals have no hidden agenda. While they can be very clever at times, their behavior is in accordance with their nature. We may think that an animal such as a tiger is devious, given that it sneaks up on its prey in order to surprise. But it is actually quite straightforward. Its prey will know from both experience and instinct that the tiger's nature is to attack in this manner. The tiger does not deviate from its natural instincts and behaviors. It is only in human beings that we primarily see devious, unpredictable, and indirect behavior.

Human beings should expect straightforwardness. This is a reflection of Nature. When we are not straightforward, we pretend, which is a kind of lying. If we develop this twisted tendency, it makes us unfit to receive right information. Māyā develops screens in our mind that lead us to develop delusions. Consequently, we will begin to interpret the information we receive from our senses incorrectly. Thus, when we act to deceive others, we will be deceived ourselves. This deception creates an imbalance in the universe. We will not see such imbalances, however, because our mind is not calm and quiet. But if we sit in meditation, we will feel disturbed by their impact.

Lack of straightforwardness—the tendency to complicate, manipulate, and distort the truth—is most often associated with a desire for money, possessions, fame, prestige, and the like. When these aims substitute as the primary goal for an individual, many problems arise due to jealousy, pride, anger, greed, and so on.

With Realization as our main goal, we will not be concerned with minor, irrelevant things. We may have a secondary aim, providing it is compatible with our primary goal, and we must approach these lesser aims in a balanced fashion, understanding that we may or may not reach them. In this way, we accept and welcome the results of karma. We must also accept that efforts in this life may or may not always yield the results we desire.

Once our primary goal of Liberation is firmly established, there will be no question of distorting our thoughts, words, or behavior. What we think, we can say. What we say, we can do. When this is possible, it brings a great amount of happiness. We will be naturally straightforward when Realization is truly our primary goal.

KṢAMĀ: RESILIENCE AND TOLERANCE

The eighth yama, *kṣamā,* means "resilience," or "tolerance and endurance." One who has kṣamā will have persistence in the face of adversity. She will have the capacity to bear disruptions with equanimity. She will show forgiveness and forbearance for the wrong actions and sins of others. When we have more kṣamā, we will naturally have more forgiveness. In Saṃskṛta, one of the names for the earth is kṣamā, because it bears all good and evil from human beings and animals. No matter what happens to it, it bears everything with a kind of silent acceptance.

The universe provides challenges for everyone. We cannot choose to rid ourselves of all challenges in life; but in the face of them, we can either lose our balance or maintain it. If we go through life without kṣamā, it is like having a hole in a dam. The more water that goes through the hole, the bigger the hole becomes and we gradually lose our capacity for kṣamā entirely. For a yoga practitioner, this would be a disaster.

If we wish to avoid being thrown off balance, we must increase kṣamā. As we look around us, we can find disruptions everywhere. Some people find challenges, no matter where they go. These people can be easily irritated by slight provocations or challenges. When we overreact to such things, we disrupt our system and our practice. It also increases our tendency to become easily irritated and develops weakness in our system.

BUILDING CAPACITY

There is a story about a *sādhaka,* or spiritual practitioner, who went on a pilgrimage to Haridwar, which is in the far north of India, near the Himalayas. The sādhaka was used to a tropical climate and wore many layers of wool clothing to protect him from the cold. One early morning, he set out for a walk and noticed a *sādhu*, or holy man, taking a bath in the freezing river. After his bath, the sādhu sat on the riverbank to do his meditation. Despite the cold, all he wore was a loincloth. The sādhaka was amazed at this and studied the sādhu for a long time. After the sādhu finished his meditation, the sādhaka approached him and asked, "Do you not feel cold?" The sādhu responded to the pilgrim, "Do you not feel cold on your face? It is exposed to the weather just as my body is!"

Naturally, we have all experienced the cold on our face, but we have developed the capacity to bear this coldness. On the other hand, we have covered our body with clothes since birth, and it has lost much of its capacity to bear the cold. As we build more and more endurance and resistance, our capacity increases; if we avoid situations that require endurance, our capacity will be reduced.

In India, domesticated elephants sometimes walk through the villages. When they do, dogs will bark at them. But even when they bark in their fiercest manner, and even when they come very close to the elephant, the elephant will not be bothered. It will not pay any attention to the dogs. It will continue to move with confidence at the same leisurely pace as if the dogs were not even there. The elephant seems to be thinking, "These dogs make irritating noises, but they do not threaten me in the slightest." This is because the elephant has a vast amount of strength when compared to a dog.

When we increase the capacity of our body and mind, we will begin to ignore small challenges and disturbances. We will understand that compared to our determination to reach the goal of Liberation, such disturbances are negligible.

It is similar to when a toddler comes up and hits us to get our attention. We may turn our attention to the child, or we may continue with whatever we happen to be doing. In either case, we will not react as though the child is beating us. Our capacity is such that we can bear the blows of the child very easily. Even if the child hits us a hundred times, we will not feel injured, whereas the child will need to sit down and rest. When we are well established in the practice of kṣamā, we will feel that the problems of this world are like the blows of the child. We will not take small problems very seriously.

DEVELOPING RESILIENCE

When the universe gives us some kind of shock or challenging situation, there are two aftereffects. The first is objective. For instance, if we cut our arm, we will feel some pain. The second is psychological. A psychological aftereffect might be thinking, "Oh, this pain is unbearable. I cannot stand it!" For the most part, the first aftereffect is not optional; we have little choice but to bear the physical pain. The second is determined by the level of reaction we have to the experience.

One person who has a stomachache may hold his abdomen and groan involuntarily. Another will not only feel the pain, but her psychological reaction may greatly amplify it. She might start fretting, "Oh, what if this pain never goes away? How can I bear it? How will I be able to do my job next week? Perhaps I have cancer! Everything always goes wrong for me!" Her psychological response is out of proportion to her physical pain.

Developing kṣamā, or resilience, will result in two significant benefits. First, it will eliminate our psychological reactions. Second, our capacity to bear the objective, physical effects will be increased significantly. These are the traits of one who has kṣamā.

We can interpret everything, including both pleasure and pain, as divine blessings. Nature only reacts against us when we have erred. This error enters our system and disturbs us. This is a kind of punishment for our error; the punishment is the medicine for the error. It is the grace of Nature to correct our errors. One who always assumes this point of view will come to enjoy all of his karma, both good and bad. Nature may create many types of problems, but one who has developed kṣamā can laugh and enjoy them all!

EQUANIMITY AND TOLERANCE

Sometimes a student will complain to a yogi about his fate. He will explain the details, elaborating on every aspect of his pain. Then he will implore the yogi, "What must I do about my karma?" The yogi might show some compassion for the student by making a few suggestions. Then, after explaining a little about kṣamā, he might suggest, "You may even learn to enjoy it!"

When we endure challenges in our life, we develop a firm balance in our system. Although there may be pain and many other disturbances, we will observe them objectively and not get attached to our psychological assessment of them. We can tolerate such suffering and experiences with equanimity.

In this way, kṣamā directly benefits our meditation practice, as well. It is impossible to ever really create a perfect place for meditation. There may be a mosquito in the room or children playing and shouting outside. It may be too hot or too cool. Maybe there is a slight ache or pain somewhere in our body. One who develops equanimity and tolerance will easily disregard all these things. She can set them aside and fully concentrate on her practice.

There is a story about a young Buddhist monk who kept complaining to his teacher about the many distractions to his meditation practice. He complained about the noise from his neighbors, from the street, and from the playground on the next block. He complained about insects and barking dogs. He complained about the smells coming from a nearby kitchen. He complained that the mornings were too cold and the evenings were too hot. He even complained about the angle of the sun as it began to bring light into his room at sunrise.

One day, after having listened patiently for several weeks, the teacher greeted the student excitedly and announced, "I have found the perfect place for you to practice. This place will solve all of your distraction problems. What do you say?" The student enthusiastically agreed. He thought that finally he would have the perfect place to practice and would easily achieve splendid yogic experiences. So the teacher gave him directions to his new meditation room. The student left the monastery and eagerly followed the directions his teacher gave him. When he arrived at the location, he discovered the teacher had secured a room for him above a busy blacksmith's shop with continuous hammers clanging and customers coming and going all day long!

The lesson for the young monk was that the ideal situation does not exist. In yoga practice, we must develop the capacity to move beyond the external distractions of our circumstances and focus on the internal.

A WISE RESPONSE

Sometimes, if we display a great deal of patience and tolerance, there will be those who try to take advantage of us. They will misuse our patience. They will intentionally misbehave in our presence, expecting that we will show patience and tolerate them. If required, we can *pretend* to lose our patience. We can scold and correct them in a measured fashion. In fact, if we do not correct them, we may be doing them a disservice. Then, even though we pretend to lose our patience, we maintain our internal balance and calm. This is skillful resistance, with compassion, toward something incorrect.

Skillful mothers know about this technique. Children inevitably misbehave. And sometimes mothers will lose their patience. But there are times, also, when a mother will feign a loss of patience. She may even shout at or scold her child. She will pretend that she is angry. She knows that the child is basically innocent and that childhood mischief is a part of growing up. Deep in her heart, she knows that the mischief is not worth losing patience over, but she will feign her reaction in order to protect and teach her child.

THE POWER OF THE MIND

How can we gain more resilience, tolerance, and equanimity? The first and most important method is by formulating a clear intention to do so. In many cases, this is enough. It will help us remember to practice such qualities. When we are aware of the benefits of kṣamā and are conscious of it becoming established within our practice, this yama will intensify. This is the nature of the mind.

The ancient legends tell us about a divine tree, the *kalpavṛkṣa,* which had the amazing quality to bestow a wish on whoever would sit under its branches and desire something. If a man wished to be a king and sit on a throne, he could depend on his wish coming true in a short time after sitting under the *kalpavṛkṣa.* This is really an allegory for the mind. When you wish for something, you may receive it immediately, or you may need to wait for it, but your wish will be fulfilled. That is why the sages encourage us to have noble wishes, such as the wish to develop kṣamā. As we develop kṣamā, we will come to appreciate and value it all the more. And the more we value it, the more it will be developed in us.

OTHER TECHNIQUES TO DEVELOP KṢAMĀ

Another technique for developing kṣamā is to associate with noble souls who demonstrate the qualities of kṣamā, like patience, tolerance, and resilience. Living near such individuals or hearing their words can automatically transmit those qualities to us.

Eating certain foods will also help us develop patience and tolerance. In general, foods like ghee, or clarified butter, and milk enrich kapha and bring endurance and patience, whereas foods that provoke vāta develop more irritation and less patience. However, kapha-dominant foods need to suit our system. If they are not suitable, though they are good foods, they can cause problems. Used incorrectly, they will cause phlegm disorders rather than developing kṣamā.

When our target is firmly fixed, we will develop ample kṣamā. If we have a serious desire and intention for Self-Realization and Liberation, we will develop a kind of detachment, or a tendency to feel equanimity toward many aspects of our life. When we are intent upon our goal, we will forget many problems and potential distractions.

If you are running late to catch a plane or train, you will focus all of your attention and energy on reaching it in time. If someone along the way shouts at you or abuses you, do you respond to them? No! You pay no attention and proceed quickly toward your gate. In the same way, having a firm spiritual goal in life helps develop kṣamā.

When we undertake the serious goal of reaching the Eternal Truth, our value system begins to change. What is the impact of some small disturbance? What is the value of this human body? What is the value of yogic achievement? What is the value of Realization of the Eternal Truth? When we contemplate these questions for ourselves, we will come to understand that small worldly disturbances are insignificant. We quickly learn to bear them easily and gracefully.

Our yoga practice develops kṣamā, and kṣamā supports our yoga practice. Because of this balance, we can more easily follow the disciplines necessary to achieve yogic experiences. We must be prepared to do whatever we need to attain Liberation. Though there will be unavoidable disturbances along the way, by being properly established in kṣamā, we may avoid being unduly distracted by them.

DHṚTI: DETERMINATION AND TENACITY

The ninth yama, *dhṛti,* is related to kṣamā. It refers to being steadfast in the face of adversity. We could call it determination with courage, or perhaps tenacity, but these are only approximate translations; there may be no equivalent English expression. In essence, the idea of dhṛti is that, once we have set our intention, it must not be disturbed by anything.

Indian scriptures tell the story of some villagers who wanted to catch a monkey and devised a simple plan. They made a small hole in a section of bamboo. The hole was just large enough for the monkey to squeeze its hand through. They then put a banana inside the hole. The monkey would see the banana, squeeze its hand through the hole, and grab hold of the banana. But with its hand now clenched into a fist, it was suddenly too large to pull back out of the hole. Given the monkey's strong determination to get the banana, even when faced with death, it would not let go. Thus, the villagers would catch the monkey, using the monkey's own determination!

SETTING INTENTION

Our determination on the path of Realization needs to be like that of the monkey. Once set, this intention should not waiver. It must be so strong that, even if we were about to die, we would not alter it. In all our lives, there will be many disturbances that tempt us to shift our intention. If there are problems, it is our duty to face them and deal with them as best we can. At the same time, we must hold our intention sacred.

Therefore, it is wise to take our time before committing to our intention. We need to make sure that our decision is sound and our goal worthy. We should look around to assess whether there might be a better goal for us. But once we make a decision, we should be steadfast in our commitment. If we often change our intention, it becomes a severe problem. If this is our tendency, we are unfit to do our spiritual practice, or *sādhana*. This fickle nature will have to be corrected before beginning serious practice.

CONFRONTING HURDLES

The spiritual journey is lifelong. It is like climbing Mount Kailasa in the Himalayas and is possible only for a person established in the practice of dhṛti. Before climbing a mountain, we must make a firm commitment to do so. On the way, we might need to cross fast-moving rivers and deep canyons. We might encounter severe weather conditions that bring rain, snow, and ice. We will succeed only if we keep our mind stable and unwavering in the face of all these obstacles. A man may have an extremely fit body and be a competent mountaineer, but if he does not possess dhṛti, he will fail. In yoga, a practitioner will face many difficulties, challenges, and even doubts along the way. With each hurdle, there will be struggle, as well as joy and wonder. None of this will hinder the practitioner who possesses dhṛti.

FEAR OF DISCONNECTION, FEAR OF DEATH

Sometimes a small child will start to cry before going to sleep. The child has been enjoying his connection to the external world and is afraid of losing the connection when he goes to sleep. In the same way, while doing his yoga practice, an aspirant may lose his connection with the external world. He may forget everything, including his family, friends, business, and all his possessions and money. This may initially cause some fear. This fear of disconnection is actually the fear of death.

Through many past lives, we have experienced death over and over again. This fear of death manifests as many other types of fears. For instance, in one birth, we may have had some fame and become attached to that fame, but death forcibly parted us from our prominence. Or we might have been very attached to our wife, husband, father, or mother. When the time came, we were forcibly separated. Fear of death is the fear of loss. Over the course of many lifetimes, we have had thousands upon thousands of experiences in which we lost the object of our attachment. This is recorded in the mind very strongly. To face loss and our fear of death requires courage.

MAINTAINING COURAGE

Some will lose courage even when grace enters their lives. If a poor man suddenly receives a large amount of money, he may lose courage as to how to manage it best. He becomes afraid of it being stolen or swindled away from him. Because of his previous lack of money, his attachment to it will be very strong. His fear of losing it will be in proportion to his attachment. A noble practitioner will have courage in the face of adversity, as well as in the presence of grace. He will maintain his balance in either case.

There was once an Indian businessman who started doing some yogic practices under the guidance of my teacher. He was extremely wealthy, even by Western standards. He was intelligent and disciplined and gained results very quickly. Then, one day, he stopped coming for instruction. He did not attend for several weeks. By chance one day, an older student of my teacher met him in the marketplace and inquired as to why he was not attending any more yoga instruction. The businessman explained that during his last practice, he had experienced a Great Light, accompanied by great joy. He became fearful that, because this joy was so attractive, he would abandon his business in favor of it. He knew that if he did that, he would lose millions of rupees. For one part of his mind, this was unbearable. So he stopped his yogic practice. This was nothing but a loss of courage.

If this man had maintained his courage, he would have discovered that the yogic experiences would have been disruptive only for a short time. After that, his mind and body would have become adjusted to them, and he would have integrated them into his daily life. After a short period of adjustment, he would have been able to maintain both his business and his yogic practice. There need not be conflict between the two. Only fear, and the lack of courage, prevented him from proceeding on his path.

When a yoga practitioner achieves certain yogic conditions, aspects of the experience will be similar to death. Her body may rest in a motionless state. She will forget the whole world, including things to which she has attachment. Her breathing may decrease dramatically or stop for a period. Her heart rate may also slow dramatically, or even stop beating entirely for a period. It is like a small death. If the practitioner is fearful about such experiences, that may prevent her from fully entering the yogic state. Her path will be blocked by that fear. This is why courage is essential. This is also why dhṛti is required to progress on the yogic path.

Dhṛti is essential for all disciplines and basic principles supporting our main intention. When one is firm in her intention, she encounters fewer and fewer obstacles. Furthermore, those obstacles that do arise will no longer be viewed as serious problems, but only as minor hindrances on the path toward one's primary goal.

MITĀHĀRA: MEASURED FOOD

Just as The *Haṭha Yoga Pradīpika,* the ancient Sanskrit manual on Haṭha Yoga, describes the tenth yama, *siddhāsana,* as the most important āsana to be practiced, it describes the tenth yama, *mitāhāra,* as the most important yama to be practiced, calling it "*yameṣuviva mitāhāra . . . rāja,*" or the kingly one among the yamas. In Saṃskṛta, *mita* means "properly measured"; *āhāra* means "food." A few have explained mitāhāra as a discipline to eat less, but that is an incorrect interpretation. To eat *measured food,* as the yama stipulates, means to eat the appropriate *amount* and *type* of food, based on our age, constitution, season, and level of activity. Even more important is that our choice of food be based on *intention,* the specific purpose that food will serve by nourishing our body. Proper use of food is the most important discipline in yoga.

But what is food? The Upaniṣads explain that this entire universe is considered to be food. Through the acts of eating, seeing, breathing, hearing, touching, and learning, we take the universe into ourselves. Āhāra, or food, includes the air that we breathe, light, sound, and even education and knowledge. All of these help our body and mind to grow. All of this, in a broad sense, is considered food. All aspects of the universe feed us, and we ourselves are food for other aspects of the universe. As our bodies decay and die, they become food for other living organisms; our actions and words may indirectly become nourishment for other beings as well. We grow from babies to adults from the food we eat. It is the food we eat that primarily constitutes our bodies. What we learn and experience feeds our minds. However, for the purpose of this book, we will focus primarily on the solid and liquid foods that serve our physical body.

We consume various types of food, and then we utilize the energy from that food. This cycle may operate properly, or it may be out of balance. When we consume the appropriate kinds and amounts of food, that is *mitāhāra*. The food will bring optimal energy to the body to support our work, our leisure activities, and our practice. When we properly and fully use that energy, our appetite will be renewed at the right time. When the time comes to eat again, our system will not contain undigested food or unused energy. Realization may be found naturally in a person who practices mitāhāra, because simple yogic techniques can work easily for him. For example, he will sit somewhere at the right time and automatically start feeling calm and quiet. At some point, this calm and quiet will be converted into meditation. Meditation will lead to Samādhi; Realization and Liberation will soon follow.

Our mind and body are the vehicles we rely on to experience Realization and Liberation. They are the products of the various foods we consume. Therefore, the consequences of consuming incorrect foods are severe. This is why it is essential to educate ourselves about the real nature of food. All yogic limbs, and sub-limbs, have some relationship to food; however, it is through mitāhāra that we will explore the subject more fully.

HONORING FOOD

There are many different species in this world. Something may be good food for one but not for another. A general principle of yoga is to never criticize any kind of food, even in our minds. There is nothing "bad" in the universe. All food is the gift of Nature. For human beings, proper food will be determined by an individual's constitution. Some food may be unsuitable for us, but suitable for others. For any type of food, there may be a person who will benefit from it.

The Indian scriptures advise against condemning even nonvegetarian food. We might not use it ourselves, but it may be a proper food for someone else's constitution. At least we can concede that this is true for animals. Certain animals would be unable to live without eating other animals. Those very animals may indirectly support our life by providing a balance in the universe. This balance may support our progression on our yogic path. For example, some bats eat mosquitoes—the troublesome insects that might otherwise bother us during our practice! We should then honor that food as well. Our task is to select food that best suits us on our yogic path.

PHYSICAL CONSTITUTIONS

Each human being has a unique constitution. In the Āyurvedic system, as mentioned earlier, there are three basic energies, sometimes called doṣas, or *dhātus,* that make up the constitution of an individual. These doṣas are vāta, pitta, and kapha and refer to the basic components of the human body. Each individual is usually a combination of two of these doṣas, with one of them having dominance; very rarely, an individual will be primarily only one doṣa or a mixture of all three.

Mitāhāra involves the proper selection of food articles based on one's doṣa, or constitution. Many people misunderstand the basic principles underlying the constitution and how best to address their imbalances. Some people have the misconception that a vāta-dominant person should avoid vāta-dominant foods, and likewise those who are pitta dominant should avoid pitta-dominant foods and those who are kapha dominant should avoid kapha-dominant foods. This is incorrect. We need to nourish the components of our constitution. This nourishment is possible only with suitable types of food. Vāta-dominant foods will nourish a vāta-dominant person, and so on.

For example, if a man is pitta-dominant, he will naturally favor pitta-dominant foods. Because his constitutional nature is to think a great deal, he will encounter many situations in life that require him to think clearly and deeply. Pitta-dominant foods will provide the proper type of energy for thinking. But even for a pitta-dominant person, there is a limit to the consumption of pitta-dominant foods. If he surpasses this limit, he will overstimulate pitta and cause disorders. He will then have difficulty practicing his meditation and yogic techniques. Pitta-dominant foods are best used in moderation.

A pitta-dominant person with a pitta-induced disease can control or eliminate the disease by reducing pitta-dominant foods for a period of time. He need not reduce his consumption of pitta-dominant foods forever. This would disturb him, because he needs the energy from those foods. To correct the disease, he should reduce those foods temporarily. If a man who is not pitta-dominant overconsumes pitta-dominant food, it will start provoking excess thoughts, which is atypical for him. As a result, he will lose sleep, and his mind will become agitated.

Those who have a complex constitution will have some of the behavior of the combined doṣas. For instance, a kapha-pitta–dominant person may pick a job as a computer programmer or writer. This job satisfies the pitta aspect of her personality: She needs to think a lot. It also satisfies the kapha aspect: She can sit calmly while working. A pitta-vāta person might make a good construction manager. Thinking about constructing a building satisfies the pitta aspect of his personality, and working hard satisfies the vāta aspect.

Ignorance about food often leads to an unhealthy condition. Most people do not really understand food or its impact. A person may simply develop a habit of eating a certain type of food, regardless of whether it supports her profession. She may be consuming too much of a particular food or eating a type that does not serve her. Unless she makes a change, her food will support neither her job nor her yoga practice.

By contrast, a fully healthy person will understand the effect of food on his body, the amount of food he requires, and the type of food that will bring the requisite energy. He will understand this inherently, not intellectually. It is a kind of intuitive insight into his body. Unfortunately, we currently live in a disturbed era. When we aim to live a more balanced way of life, we will understand food and its influence on our body. Our entire relationship to food will change. We will live in accordance with these new principles.

NONVEGETARIANISM

No food is unequivocally bad. For each type of food, someone or something will benefit from eating it. For instance, not all human beings are meant to be vegetarians. This is true all over the world, including in India. If someone who is not a vegetarian wants to practice yoga, what must they do? Must they stop eating all nonvegetarian food?

There are two types of practitioners. Some go slowly, according to their own nature; they will move deliberately toward Liberation. Others will feel an internal drive to move very quickly toward that goal.

Those who are by birth nonvegetarians and want to proceed toward Liberation at a gradual pace may use nonvegetarian food. However, they will feel some disturbances. They will need to face those disturbances and resolve them through suitable remedies. Any food that we consume requires corresponding activities to burn the energy that it provides. If a practitioner eats nonvegetarian food, he should select a job that makes maximum use of that energy. Then, even though he is consuming nonvegetarian food, he may still reach the final target. A serious practitioner should eat only vegetarian food, however. Compared to nonvegetarian food, it will offer more support in keeping the mind calm and quiet.

The great epics of India—the Mahābhārata and the Rāmāyaṇa—include examples of yogic personalities consuming nonvegetarian food. Such incidents are either exceptions or appropriate only for that particular era. Thousands of years ago, the digestive fire for human beings was much more responsive to the power of intention. However, as the times have changed, the digestive fire of all human beings has gradually lost much of its original capacity. Today, only sattvic food can be digested for sattvic purposes. We should not justify our own unfavorable food habits by citing these ancient examples.

When a person has a very strong digestive fire, she can consume and easily digest many different types of foods, including very spicy food, and even certain other unsuitable foods. However, an ill person will be very disturbed by mildly spicy or heavy food; this will interfere with her well-being.

In India, the *kṣatriya* caste is the traditional caste of warriors and kings. Members of that caste ate nonvegetarian food, and some of those souls were Realized. However, when kṣatriyas began to practice yoga seriously, they followed the vegetarian principle.

In addition to the problems of digestion, and conversion of food to sattvic energy, there is another consideration regarding nonvegetarian food. Yogis place a great deal of emphasis on nonviolence. Even though there is a certain amount of violence involved in eating vegetables, yogis recommend vegetarian food. As we explained in the section on the yama ahimsā, animals have a greater capacity for happiness than vegetables do. Moreover, there is greater life activity in animals than in vegetation. It is common sense to support life where it is seen more vividly. We can allow and encourage happiness in these highly sentient forms of life. If we let animals live so that they can enjoy more happiness, we are doing less harm. Even in ancient days, many lived by this principle, and it is still valid today.

As the great sage Manu tells us, "There is nothing bad in eating nonvegetarian food, nor in drinking alcohol, nor sexual activity within a committed relationship. These are natural tendencies for all human beings. But those who control these three will receive the most wonderful results in their yogic practice."

We receive more strength in the body if we eat nonvegetarian food. But how much physical strength do we need for our occupation? A soldier needs a lot of strength. A yoga practitioner does not need that much. We will select the quantity, quality, and type of food we eat based on our needs. For Realization and Liberation, we need to consider not only *how much* energy we need, but also what *type* of energy we need. We need to decide these things in a thoughtful, careful way.

HOW KARMA AND SAṂSKĀRA AFFECT WHAT WE EAT

The energy from food is energy for both our body and our mind. We desire and consume foods that move us on a course according to our karmas and saṃskāras. These need to play out and bring their results. Different types of food will support different types of karma and saṃskāra. Thus, a particular saṃskāra will provoke the mind to desire a particular type of food whose energy will support that saṃskāra to manifest.

This is not to suggest that we may necessarily reverse our fate by forcibly changing the foods we eat. To a large extent, Nature has laid out the course of our lives at the time of conception. Nature decides many factors at that time, including our gender and our constitution. Though it is all but impossible to change either of these two aspects, our interests and aptitudes—which drive our education and occupation in life—are influenced by our previous lives and will be played out through our karmas and saṃskāras.

FOOD NEEDS ACCORDING TO CAREER

Each individual needs different types and quantities of energy for their body and mind, depending on their profession, activities, and, to some extent, the climate in which they live. A teacher requires different food than a soldier. A manual laborer needs one type and quantity of food, whereas office personnel have different requirements. A construction worker needs to eat food that supports physical strength. A man who needs to sit calmly and quietly will gain strength and stability from dairy products. A woman with a highly intellectual job, requiring her to think deeply, needs more pungent and spicy foods, as these foods will provoke thoughts. Based on the integrated knowledge of yoga and Āyurveda, the type of work we do, as well as the climate we live in, determines which foods we need to eat.

Ideally, our profession will be aligned with our constitution. If we pick a job that is unsuitable for us, we will struggle in our work. This is a widespread problem in the world these days. Many people choose a profession based on how much money they expect to earn rather than what is suitable for them. They do not consider which job will offer them the most happiness and contentment. This is mostly because they confuse the money they will earn with the happiness they seek. Sometimes a person will select an unsuitable job because of some karma from a previous birth. In that case, the job requires one type of food and the person's constitution requires another. If this person eats food that supports his profession, it will not nourish his constitution; if he eats food that supports his constitution, it will not nourish his profession. Moreover, he will not excel at his job but will do only an adequate or a mediocre job. The type of work we do needs to be compatible with our system. Therefore, we should be very careful in selecting our career. If there is some karma that prevents us from choosing wisely, we must seek the advice of a knowledgable yogi or Āyurvedic doctor to help guide us.

If our job suits our system, then our job itself will be yoga. Our work will bring balance to our system. It will support our Realization. What is yoga, really? It is nothing but a balance in our system that allows us to eventually reach yogic states. When the job is suitable for our constitution, it is easier to decide which food will support us.

Proper food and right livelihood are closely connected. Today there are many problems associated with both. We see many people employed in poorly chosen occupations who, in addition, have no idea about what kind of food they should be eating. They select food that is not meant for their constitution. Many people in a society will eat the same food, though it will not be beneficial to all in the same way. Each person should adjust his eating habits to his particular needs. Certainly, there will be some common foods all people share, but there will also be some meaningful differences, as each individual is unique.

FOOD AND INTENTION

If we can find our primary intention in life, we will be able to select foods that support it. We can see that a bird is not suited to pull an oxcart, and that a snake is not at home in a swimming pool. Similarly, we can examine ourselves and see if Nature has already determined our main intention. We can identify our own constitution. We can assess the capabilities of our body and mind, including which are the most powerful. And finally, we can ask the most important question of all: What is the real intention of this human body? Once we understand Nature's intention in creating human beings, it will be easier to act in accordance with that intention.

For example, while attending college, our primary intention might be to secure an appropriate position after graduation. Our secondary intention may include graduating with good grades, working at a part-time job that helps support us financially while we are in school, and having good friendships and meeting knowledgeable teachers.

Throughout life, we make these choices, consciously or unconsciously. One will have musical talents and decide to become a singer; another will become an artist, writer, college professor, or doctor. The guiding principle in deciding our intention in life is that it should not hinder our progress toward Realization and Liberation. Our professions, or interests, should never be a deviation from this primary goal. A singer will gain enormous support for Liberation through devotional chanting or songs that encourage the highest ideals in humankind. A writer may use her skills to educate others about life and receive support through her writing. In this way, each honorable occupation helps steer us toward our primary goal. Likewise, our diet should support our constitution, and thereby our intentions in life.

HOW MUCH TO EAT?

One of the biggest hindrances for human beings in reaching their primary intention is overconsumption of food. Traditionally, in India, two different units of measure are used to determine the optimal quantity of food to ingest. The first is a way to determine when we have eaten enough. This measurement is based on an individual's stomach capacity. Yogic texts recommend that at each meal we eat only enough solid food to fill half of our stomach; we drink enough liquid food (this may be water or soup) to fill one fourth; the remaining fourth we leave for air to ensure proper digestion. This means that we develop the discipline to stop eating when we feel that we could eat half as much food again. This also requires self-awareness and a kind of introspective view into our own body to understand how much food we have eaten and the capacity of our stomach.

This method of measuring food will only work for a person who has a balanced mind. If we are upset, if we have much strain and tension in our system, or if we are undisciplined, this method will not be successful. Many try to relax their minds through eating. This often leads to overeating. Our stomachs are made out of muscles and membranes. They are flexible. When our stomach is consistently stretched to accommodate overeating, it will gain more and more capacity. In such cases, this method of measurement no longer works. However, a man with a balanced mind will understand how much food he has eaten. He has the capacity to understand when his stomach is filled to the proper extent. He also has the discipline to stop eating at the appropriate time.

Another traditional method of measuring food is based on the number of *mouthfuls* eaten. The size of a person's hand will be roughly proportionate to the overall size of that individual's body. Thus, the amount of food that one picks up in her hand is meaningful. A large man will naturally pick up more food than a small woman. A child will pick up an even smaller amount. In the West, we may equate this amount roughly with one spoonful or forkful of food. Naturally, this is not equivalent to using one's hand because it will not adjust for the size of the person. An alternative is to base this measurement on one comfortable mouthful of food.

A male or female householder between the ages of twenty-four and sixty, who is not working very hard, will need to consume thirty-two mouthfuls of food twice a day. If this person is working very hard for many hours each day, this should be expanded a little bit—not by eating more at one meal, but by adding another small meal in the morning, perhaps of sixteen mouthfuls of food.

You can simply test this. While eating a meal, count your mouthfuls and see if thirty-two mouthfuls of food are adequate for you. In order to better assess how your body feels, it is best to eat in silence when you do this experiment. Eating without talking will help you to objectively assess your body and prevent strain on your digestion.

CHILDREN AND FOOD

There is no restriction on the quantity of food for a youth who is involved in a rigorous yogic education and performs daily yogic practices. Children can eat however much is required to maintain a growing body and an expanding mind, though each person will need a different amount of food, according to body structure. One person may be short. Another may be tall and lean. A third may be tall with a strong, stout body. During this period of growth, people will vary widely as to how much food they need. In general, a growing student can use as much as needed.

However, young people who have problems with family or peers may develop unhealthy psychological conditions that cause them to overeat or even undereat. This may also arise due to karma and saṃskāra from previous births. When this overeating behavior occurs, a competent teacher, supervisor, or parent should educate and offer suggestions. Such young people have lost the ability to measure their own food correctly. Someone must guide them with compassion and understanding. They should be given some meaningful information about food and how much they should consume. Most important, they should be helped with any underlying psychological disturbances.

When a father and mother provide good role models, children will generally be very healthy. When a child lives in a family where parents love each other, and love their children, all members will be naturally healthy. The child's mind will be calm and quiet. In general, these children will be satisfied with their lives. If that healthy child goes to a well-managed school, he will experience even more inner calm and quiet. A child like this will not crave excess food and will naturally limit his food consumption.

THE ELDERLY AND FOOD

Elderly people need less food than others. In India, those who were older than sixty would traditionally go to live in a forest or an isolated place. There they had only a few light duties to care for, so they were free to concentrate fully on yoga and Liberation. Someone of that age, and with that simple way of life, would consume only sixteen mouthfuls of food at a sitting, twice per day. However, this is no longer a common practice today.

A few very serious practitioners will not live the typical life of a householder. Their sole goal in life is Liberation. Some of these individuals will follow a practice of maintaining *silence*. Such a person is called a *muni*. This is mostly because talking takes energy, and energy requires us to consume more food. A muni does not talk, so he does not need much food. He may need to eat only eight mouthfuls of food per meal, twice a day. This is enough for him to maintain his body in order to practice his yoga.

FOOD FOR BRAHMACĀRIS AND MONKS

With few exceptions, all types of sattvic food will suit brahmacāris and monks. Monks should eat only one meal at midday and a small snack in the evening. Since a brahmacāri is still in his youth and his body growing, he may eat two meals and a snack, depending upon his particular need. It is also recommended that monks generally eat alone—a practice that a common person should try to avoid. There are also various food restrictions that monks and brahmacāris should recognize. For example, the Indian tradition of eating *betel leaf* after a meal is not recommended, as it slightly provokes sexual tendencies.

LISTENING TO THE BODY

The best way to measure food is simply by intuitively becoming aware of your body's response to eating. A healthy human being will feel some signs from her body when she has consumed adequate food. As she is eating, at some point, she will feel, "This is enough. I do not require any more." That is the point at which to stop eating. Healthy children easily demonstrate this capability. After a child has eaten a sufficient quantity of food, she will refuse another spoonful. But, over time, many of us stop paying attention to these signs from our bodies and lose the ability to recognize them. After we become established in mitāhāra, we regain this capacity.

FOOD AND ILLNESS

When we follow the discipline of mitāhāra, we will end up with a balanced mind. Conversely, one with a balanced mind will naturally consume the proper type and amount of food. Whenever we treat a disease or imbalance, we should always treat it from two directions.

First, we look at the cause of the illness in the mind. Why is the mind creating imbalance? What is the remedy to effectively treat the mind? Second, we treat it by correcting factors in the external world—namely, by paying attention to the type and amount of food we are consuming. In this way, we tackle the imbalance from both an internal and external approach.

These days, a psychologist might attempt to treat a problem through the mind alone. A physician might attempt to treat the problem only on the physical level. A more comprehensive treatment will address the problem on both the physical and mental levels. If we tackle our problems from both directions, we can solve them more easily.

THE INFLUENCE OF OUR BIRTHPLACE ON OUR CONSTITUTIONS

When we eat in a more natural way, our system will become more calm and quiet. One of the principles of eating in a more natural way is to eat the foods that are grown in the region where we were born. There is a meaningful link between our birthplace and our bodies. The vegetation grown in that area will be more suitable for our constitution. In general, we will find it easier to digest and more satisfying. We will also find that it gives us the proper type of energy for our activities. Our birthplace is extremely important and deserves to be honored. In days past, the system of choosing food worked very naturally. People did not travel much. Many would spend their entire lives near where they were born. The food of that area was very suitable and natural to them.

However, these days this method of selecting food is not practical. Systems of commerce distribute foods all around the world for consumption. Of course, this is sometimes essential to feed large populations of people living far from the gardens and fields where food is grown.

This principle is also disturbed by our tendency to travel the world over and to easily change the place we live. Many people live far away from their birthplace because they are seeking work opportunities, educational opportunities, or simply desiring different lifestyles from their parents. We can hop on a plane and be on the other side of the world in one day. Within our own country, we move from here to there simply to visit friends or engage in leisure activities. As a result, many people lose the potential benefit that the food from their birthplace may provide their systems.

The next principle is that food grown close to our current residence is better for us than food that is shipped over a long distance. If we live in a cold, northern climate, wheat and potatoes will provide warmth. If we live in a tropical climate, rice and lighter vegetables are easier to digest. Predominance should be given to food from our birthplace for the major portion of the food that we eat. And, of course, it is much more practical and beneficial for the environment, instead of shipping foods long distances with the use of fossil fuels.

To some extent we can adjust our diet to accommodate both our birthplace and the place where we currently live. If we were born in a cold climate but are currently living in a tropical area, we will naturally eat more wheat than someone who has lived in a tropical climate since birth. The opposite will be true, also. One who was born in a tropical climate but moved to a cold climate will consume more rice than someone native to the cold climate. If we have radically changed our place of habitation, we will have one food as the major source of nutrition and another food as a minor source of nutrition. The major food will be chosen based on where we were born and the minor food based on where we live.

Even though they may not be grown everywhere, some foods are nonetheless useful for humankind in small proportions. For example, if raisins are not grown where we live, it does not hurt us to use some for variety. Saffron is grown only in a very few parts of the world, but everyone can use it. It does not cause any problem; it is a beneficial food. There are many such examples from all over the world. Unlike the haphazard introduction of foods into our diet today, these foods have been discovered through yogic sight, and their benefits closely observed by yogis and through the science of Āyurveda for generations to determine their acceptability and usefulness in our diet. However, we should still give priority to food originating from our birthplace, which will have a major influence on our whole body and be the most compatible for our systems.

The epic poem the Rāmāyaṇa says that our birthplace is like heaven. In the poem, a *rākṣasa,* or demon, named Rāvaṇa kidnaps the noble Rāma's wife, Sītā and takes her to his home in Sri Lanka, an exceptionally beautiful country with much wealth and delicious food. Near the end of the epic, Rāma and his brother, Lakṣmaṇa, are engaged in a lively discussion. Lakṣmaṇa expounds on the beauty of Sri Lanka and enthusiastically says to Rāma, "This place is glorious. Why should we not live here?" Rāma immediately responds, "Our mother and our birthplace are like heaven. We should not forget either one. That place alone brings full harmony to our system. Let the brother of Rāvaṇa live here. This is his birthplace, and it suits him. He will rule this kingdom wisely, but we must return to Ayodhya. That is our birthplace."

If we change the place where we live and dwell there for at least twelve years, we will see a radical change in our system. This is the time it takes for our system, mind and body, to change at the root level. Although we can sometimes make minor changes quickly, to change something at the systemic level takes much longer. After twelve years, we will find that the food grown where we live, rather than where we were born, will have become more suitable.

Where we live has a big influence on the food we select, and the food we eat has a tremendous effect on our yogic pursuits. If we are dedicated to a yoga practice, we need to let our practice play a major role in deciding where we will live. There are places in this world for many kinds of creatures. Some places will be very suitable to specific varieties of plants and animals. Certain birds will naturally live in a cold environment, and other species will live in a tropical area. Some animals must live in a polar region. If we try to move them to a warmer place, they will die. Each creature will receive suitable support from the plants and vegetation that grow in the area where it lives. Human beings can live in a polar region, but then they will normally consume ample quantities of meat for the warmth and strength it provides. But is such a place good for a yoga practitioner? A practitioner needs a great deal of calm and balanced energy in his system. This energy helps the mind move inward.

THE THREE BASIC ENERGIES AND FOOD

As we saw earlier, there are three basic energies in the universe called guṇas—specifically, sattva, rajas, and tamas. Each of these three will be dominant in our system at different periods of the day. Each appropriately supports different activities in our life. When tamas is dominant, it supports our sleep. Rajas wakes us from sleep and provides energy for our extroverted activities, such as our profession. When sattva dominates, it helps to focus and calm our mind and body and, ultimately, brings about yogic experiences. To progress on the yogic path, sattva must be the dominant energy in our system. This is made possible only by eating sattvic food. But what is sattvic food?

Over the ages, yogis have analyzed many varieties of food and determined their intrinsic qualities. Each variety will be partly sattvic, rajasic, and tamasic; it will have a certain balance of these three basic energies. Some foods, such as milk and ghee, are inherently sattvic. They have a naturally calming effect. Other foods, such as onions and garlic, are inherently rajasic. They cause vigilance, and their influence will allow us to attend to many duties at once. They also increase the activity in the mind. They are good for a soldier or farmer but hinder meditation practice. Still other foods, such as mushrooms, are predominantly tamasic. If we eat enough of them, we will feel sleepy. Tamasic foods may disturb our rajasic activities, such as our professional work, and our sattvic activities, including meditation. To the extent that the main quality of a food is sattvic, it will help our meditation. If the main quality is rajasic or tamasic, it will hinder our meditation; therefore, yoga practitioners do best to avoid such foods.

Beyond the inherent characteristics of food, the properties of foods will change based on the way we prepare and combine them. Certain combinations of food provoke tamas. If we mix yogurt with a dish using black *gram dhal*, it becomes tamasic and will provoke sleep. Or if we prepare and store food for some time before consuming it, the food becomes tamasic. This is one reason that it is best to eat freshly prepared food.

OTHER INFLUENCING FACTORS

There are many important aspects related to how we consume our food. Our state of mind while preparing and eating our meals has a considerable effect on the food that we eat. Other influencing factors include where we eat, with whom we eat, and what else we may be doing at the time. All these things have an impact on the food we eat and how it ultimately serves us. A serious practitioner will follow many disciplines, so that food will support his yogic practice.

The way we get our food is also very important. If violence has been involved, it will have a negative impact on us. For example, we can purchase and prepare very sattvic food items, such as milk, ghee, and rice, but if the money used to buy this food was stolen, the food will have a strong rajasic and tamasic effect on us.

VARIOUS FOODS AND THEIR PROPERTIES

Food can be either a tremendous support or a major hindrance to our yogic practice. The Bhagavad-Gītā offers the advice "For one who eats right food, yoga eliminates all types of misery." In another stanza it warns, "One who eats too much cannot attain yoga."

In general, it is best for a yoga practitioner to eat grains, legumes, fresh vegetables, and fruits. The best foods for yogic practice are sattvic foods and will be naturally sweet. This does not mean that the foods contain refined sugar. Rice and wheat have a natural sweetness, as do carrots and many other fruits and vegetables. Some of the more common sattvic foods are rice, wheat, barley, ghee, milk, buttermilk, honey, jaggery (unrefined cane sugar), ginger, some gourds and squashes, and some leafy vegetables. Prepared dishes may also include a little bit of fat, such as ghee or oil. Sesame oil, peanut oil, olive oil, and other vegetable oils are all suitable.

Legumes, such as mung beans and mung *dhal,* are very favorable for yogic practice; *toor dhal* and *bengal gram dhal* are also acceptable. Black gram dhal is satisfactory if used in moderation. If used too much, it provokes tamas, and if used with yogurt, it provokes even more tamas. Black beans and pinto beans bring much energy to the body but can create vāta imbalance and cause joint pain. Those who work hard physically can more easily tolerate these foods; they will also support the body for hard work.

Most of the fruits that are not totally sour are excellent for yoga practice. Each fruit has its own unique nature. Some fruits, such as papaya and mango, should be consumed with milk. Some sour fruits, such as gooseberry, can be consumed with jaggery, raw sugar, or honey. Mixing the fruit with raw sugar or honey will eliminate the negative qualities due to the sour taste. Pomegranate, if of good quality, is especially beneficial for yogic practice. When overripe, most fruits are considered tamasic and should not be eaten.

Apples are generally a sattvic food but might need to be peeled before eating for those who find the skin hard to digest. The skin of the guava fruit is easy to digest, but the seeds are best discarded for digestive purposes.

Most gourds are sattvic and support yoga practice. In India, the ash gourd is the king of vegetables, but it may not be available in all parts of the world. It is nourishing, easy to digest, and very sattvic. Many squashes are in this category. The cucumber is harmless. It does not give much strength. It contains a lot of water and is a light, easily digestible food. Some people who are unable to undertake a total fast because of health problems can eat this type of food during a fast.

Almost all vegetables may be used freely, although a few are rajasic and a few tamasic. *Palak* is a leafy vegetable similar to spinach found in India. Both palak and spinach have a tamasic effect.

Many root vegetables, such as carrots and beets, are good for yogic practice. Potatoes are fine in moderation, although they can be heavy on the digestion, causing gas and bloating. Those who have a tendency toward a bulky body should use them very sparingly. Sweet potatoes and yams are also heavy to digest, so it is better to use them sparingly, or mix them with pepper or ginger to reduce the heaviness. The smell of the radish hinders yogic practice; however, the radish contains medicinal properties. Those who have piles or constipation benefit from radishes. Sometimes those who wish to eat radishes will peel, cook, and rinse them, which eliminates much of the smell.

If possible, it is better to select organic foods that have been raised naturally, without pesticides or chemical fertilizers. Sometimes such foods are not available, or are too expensive, so there is no other option. We have to eat what is available.

Coffee creates a great deal of mental disturbance. As a stimulant, it provokes thoughts and hinders yoga practice. It disturbs the whole mood of meditation. Even if one drinks coffee after concluding yoga practice, it disrupts the results. Tea is not as bad, but it still disturbs. These drinks will reduce appetite and, when consumed regularly over time, will reduce the effectiveness of many Āyurvedic medicines.

EATING SEASONALLY

Proper food selection is also based on the season. In winter or during the cold times of the year, heavy foods keep the body warm and are thus beneficial. In the summer, the same foods are heavy for the body and disturb meditation. Sweeter foods keep the body cool and support meditation. As indicated by Āyurveda, it is best to start to change food types about two weeks before the season's change. If we gradually change food slightly from one season to the next, it will help our body maintain balance.

The availability of foods differs drastically from one part of the world to another. We should look around us in our own country, state, and city and determine what food items are available. Then, from those options, we select what will best suit our intentions. We do what is possible and make our best efforts given our circumstances.

QUALITY OF FOOD

We should seek food with maximum health-giving qualities. To do so, we must understand the potentially beneficial and harmful properties associated with the food we eat. It is difficult to find high-quality food today for many reasons.

For example, milk today is typically of poor quality. It is a whitish liquid that may look like milk, but it does not have the properties that we expect. First of all, cows these days are crossbreeds, bred only for the quantity of milk they produce. As a result, they are unhealthy animals with both visible and invisible imbalances in their systems. The properties of the milk obtained from naturally bred cows are lost in crossbreeds. If we taste the milk of the original breeds of cows, it will be sweet even without sugar. It will affect the body and mind in very beneficial ways. Previously, milk was used for the very specific purpose of aiding humankind in Liberation. That purpose is no longer being served. We simply cannot compare the impact of that milk to the milk that we purchase today.

Although grapes and raisins are considered among the best fruits to eat, according to Āyurveda, even many Western scientists are concerned about the negative impact from chemicals used in growing grapes. Similarly, the use of pesticides in growing potatoes, carrots, and sweet potatoes add poisons to our body. We are even more susceptible when eating leafy vegetables like cabbage, lettuce, and kale, whose leaves easily absorb pesticides. An alternative is to purchase and consume organically grown food, but this only partially addresses the problem.

Today there are large imbalances in the overall natural ecology of the earth. Yoga says that the root of this problem is due to a loss of *dharma* throughout the world. In Indian philosophy and literature, *dharma* primarily refers to Brahma, the seed for this entire universe, the Eternal Truth. In a secondary sense, dharma is the right condition in which the Eternal Truth best offers its presence in the world. It is also *right action* that sustains this healthy condition. This includes properly using materials in this world—living and nonliving—so as to create optimal conditions for the presence of the Eternal Truth. Dharma is what keeps everything in this world in total health and balance. The loss of dharma is what has upset the natural order. Hence, we see excess growth of pests and blight that destroy food crops. Rather than attacking these creatures, however, we can begin to address this problem by maintaining the principles of Nature. Only by properly understanding the role of dharma will we heal the planet.

ENJOYMENT OF FOOD

We can taste six flavors in food: sweet, salty, sour, spicy, bitter, and astringent. Although some traditional Indian recipes have only four or five of these flavors, most traditional Indian preparations blend all six flavors. Food prepared with all six will be very satisfying and supportive to yoga practice.

Eating food that tastes good to us is very important. Otherwise, we will not feel satisfied with our meal. The feeling of satisfaction brings balance to many emotions that are essential to a healthy human being. If we consume food that does not have the proper taste, there will be something lacking in our emotional state. Balanced emotions support us to enjoy both bhoga and yoga.

Eating proper and delicious food is very important for an aspirant. It is our duty to eat correctly. It is also our duty to know how to prepare sattvic food. We need not be gourmet vegetarian cooks, but at the very least, we should be able to prepare nutritious, tasty food that will support our yogic practice.

FOOD PREPARATION

Cooking is one of the sixty-four traditional Indian yogic sciences, or paths for Realization. The cook is expected to follow certain disciplines while preparing food. The mindset of the cook deeply affects the food. If food is prepared by someone who is agitated, impatient, greedy, or overly sexual, those qualities will to some degree be transmitted through the food to those who eat it.

This idea may seem foreign to some people. They are in the habit of eating whatever food is offered, no matter who prepares it. They do not take into account the mentality of the person cooking their food.

Within India, the cook's mindset is considered to be extremely significant. The members of some yogic circles will eat only food prepared by someone within their group. For many, there will be no exception to this rule.

It is important for the person preparing the food to remain as calm and quiet as possible. If one looks at food, directly or indirectly, one's influence is transferred to the food in a way similar to touching it. In addition to maintaining a calm and quiet demeanor, thinking about divine subjects is also highly beneficial while preparing food. If the cook is a seeker of Truth, holding the thought that her efforts to prepare the meal will support aspirants will also have a very positive effect. Food prepared in this fashion will have an added benefit. If the quality of the raw food, the mindset of the cook, the method of preparation, and the approach of the one eating the food are all in accordance with yogic principles, the food will bring a wonderful balance to the body.

A generous attitude on the part of the cook is most important. One should never feel that there is not enough food to serve others. Cooking should not be a burden; it is best approached as a privileged task in which one takes pleasure. The cook is in fact serving humankind and helping others on the journey toward the Eternal Truth. It is an honor to be the cook and to support others by preparing good food for them.

It is also best not to think about eating while preparing food. If the cook looks at the food eagerly, thinking that it will be delicious, the food will not bring optimal results. There are certain disciplines related to this principle. In general, the cook should not taste the food while cooking. However, when one is learning how to cook, this discipline may be relaxed a bit. Cooking without tasting is a difficult task for a beginner.

If the cook enjoys singing, then singing some *bhajans,* or other devotional songs, supports food preparation by helping the cook maintain a calm mind. Singing also has a directly favorable impact on the food.

INFLUENCE OF THE KITCHEN

We have already learned that foods are predominantly sattvic, rajasic, or tamasic. Also, we have discussed the many ways that food may gain or lose certain qualities and how the methods by which we prepare foods can change their basic guṇa energy. To this end, the kitchen must be kept pure, clean, and free from all detrimental energetic influences. After all, the place where we cook precious food to nourish this priceless human body is sacred.

CHANGE DUE TO COOKING

Even though we can objectively classify any food as predominantly sattvic, rajasic, or tamasic by nature, the method of preparation can change the dominant guṇa, or energy of that food. Preparation can transform a sattvic quality of a food into rajasic or tamasic qualities. When we combine various unprocessed food ingredients, it produces an effect like a chemical reaction. The result of the recipe is not just the sum of the parts. The cooked food has a set of properties all its own. Those new properties may or may not be favorable to our health and yogic practice. Depending on the method of preparation, a few foods become tamasic. Similarly, a few become sattvic. In Saṃskṛta, this changing of the properties of food due to cooking is called *pāka*. We can understand this with a simple example. Raw, hot chilies provoke pitta. They are far too hot for many people to eat. However, frying chilies in ghee reduces their heat by half, and combining the fried chilies with yogurt reduces their heat by half again.

One of the most important principles in yogic cooking requires that we eat the food soon after it is cooked. If we store the cooked food too long, it becomes tamasic. This influence starts well before the food becomes "spoiled." In particular, steamed rice must be eaten within three hours. In general, all cooked food should be consumed within three hours of being prepared. Its nature changes drastically after that point. A yoga practitioner whose body and mind are in optimal balance will easily understand this. After eating cooked food that has been kept for several hours, he will feel a type of sleepiness or drowsiness. Moreover, all tamasic foods are difficult to digest.

Some foods, because of the method of their preparation, will last for a much longer time. Some fried Indian snacks will last for weeks. Of course, these foods should not be eaten as the main food. They are to be used sparingly. Chapatis (unleavened bread) will last for many hours if we prepare them with less oil or ghee and cook them until they are fully dry. As such, they make good travel food.

STORAGE AND REHEATING

Any food that is reheated becomes tamasic. Keeping food in the refrigerator until the next day and then heating it in the microwave oven does not have a favorable impact on it. In fact, cooking food twice doubles its tamasic quality. Making toast out of bread is an example of this. It is better to eat bread without toasting it. Refried beans are another example.

If it becomes absolutely necessary to keep food in the refrigerator, it is better to consume the food immediately after removing it—even if one wishes to reheat it slightly. Otherwise, its tamasic qualities will quickly increase. The refrigeration restricts the conversion to tamasic food, but when the saved food is removed from the refrigerator and placed in the open, its tamasic qualities increase much faster than the increase in tamas after cooking food.

In the West particularly, many people have jobs that allow them little time during the week to prepare food properly. They feel they must either eat at a restaurant or prepare food ahead of time and refrigerate or freeze it for later use. Many problems result from eating restaurant food. We do not know about the quality of the ingredients or how it was prepared. Sometimes the food is reheated many times. We have no way of knowing the mindset or the level of hygiene of the people preparing the food. These factors will all affect us when we eat this food. What to do when we have no time to cook becomes a matter of picking the solution that causes the fewest problems. Eating our own food that has been kept in the refrigerator or freezer is better than eating restaurant food.

One positive use of the refrigerator is for the storage of vegetables, seeds, and other raw foods. In today's society, it is impossible for most of us to go to the field or forest every day to collect our vegetables. We must purchase them and sometimes keep them for several days. Storing uncooked food in the refrigerator has almost no negative impact.

A very natural lifestyle in which we could collect fresh vegetables every day would be even more ideal, however. Growing a small garden can serve that purpose to some degree. There are also many other benefits one may experience from having a small garden. For example, one may gain beneficial exercise, as well as deep satisfaction in doing garden work. If done in a measured and relaxed way, it may lead to a calm and quiet mind.

COOKING AS A SACRED DUTY

Cooking, according to the disciplines of a yogic way of life, is a full-time job. Previously, this was the tradition in India. However, today men and women are overly attached to making money. They find a job and work extremely hard to earn as much money as possible. They are not available in their home to support a yogic lifestyle. If a man has this approach to money, chances are his wife will also share these feelings. She too may feel it necessary to find a job and earn more money. In such a case, the home and kitchen may start to seem like a prison. Some women feel that it is a form of discrimination for her husband to have a career while she stays at home to attend to such duties.

In a more traditional situation, it was common for the husband to seek a proper livelihood that allows him to spend ample time at home doing yogic practices, so then his wife might feel that it is a pleasure to stay at home and prepare food that supports their yogic paths. She would understand that this is an extremely important aspect of yoga practice and would consider it an honor and privilege to engage in such meaningful activity. She would fully enjoy studying the yogic science of cooking. She would understand how food preparation affects the mind. She would become a partner in the household's common journey toward Realization and Liberation.

When we devote ourselves to yogic practice, the preparation of food cannot be a part-time job. It requires a vast amount of time and is best done in a relaxed and calm atmosphere. If both spouses have jobs outside the home, as is very common in contemporary society, it is unlikely there will be enough time for any one person to do the cooking correctly and each spouse will always be hurried.

Though it may seem controversial when read through a modern lens, the traditional teachings say that working outside the home disturbs a woman's constitution. Qualities such patience, nurturance, and softness can be more easily depleted outside the home. Knowledge and practice of the principles of cooking brings much spontaneous joy. If a husband properly understands his relationship to his own work and yoga, he will fully support his wife's pursuit of traditional duties. When both spouses are engaged with pursuing their traditional, rightful duties, the entire family will grow in a spiritual direction and develop a healthy mentality.

Moreover, the best teaching that a mother can offer her children is to feed them properly. By doing so, she will be able to influence her children in the best possible manner. Naturally, her words will also support them, but her most effective form of teaching is through her food. Feeding them is not simply a matter of putting food with sufficient nourishment before them. By example, she teaches her children about the importance and meaningfulness of food on the yogic path. She imparts the principles of food selection and preparation, as well as those related to consuming it. This is the true meaning of feeding her children.

Family life, in India and all over the world, has become twisted. Today a career as a homemaker can make a woman feel like a second-class citizen. In reality, she has a highly honored position in the home and will be loved very much by all who understand this. She deserves to be revered like a deity. She should be fully supported in her work by all the others in the home, because she is the one who provides precious food. Without that precious food, the others in the home cannot progress on their yogic path, so they fully honor her. This tradition is rapidly slipping away.

While implementing or reclaiming these traditional gender roles is not realistic for many modern practitioners, understanding the roots of these teachings is invaluable. The essences of the teachings may resonate with practitioners on different levels.

GUESTS

When hungry guests arrive at our home, it is our duty to offer them food. If we are eating a meal, and someone nearby is craving food, his craving will have an adverse effect on us. In general, it is better to share our food with those around us. In India, if anybody arrives at mealtime, it is a cause for celebration, a festival of sorts. Feeding guests is considered an honor. There is a tradition still practiced in small villages today in which a man will meet the midday bus and look for a guest to invite to his home for the midday meal. The host's extension of hospitality to his guest is viewed as having a positive influence on his home.

THE ACT OF EATING

Once food is purchased or collected, washed and prepared, we eat it. The way we eat the food is another important factor that determines its influence on our body. Our attitude and thoughts when we eat have a critical effect on the food. It is best to have a calm and quiet mind and to remember the reason that we are eating the food, which is to achieve Realization. To emphasize this aspect, chanting some prayers before eating is a common practice that adds the impact of sound. The purpose of chanting is to strengthen the ideal thought "I am using this food, which is a gift of Nature. Let this food serve my Liberation. Let this food bring a right mind, right body, and suitable strength." There is a tradition of saying a short prayer before eating. In doing so, we acknowledge that the food belongs to Nature and supports us in our quest for nonattachment and Liberation: "To earn food one should do justified work. One should eat food to sustain one's prāṇa. Prāṇas are to be nourished to know the cosmic Truth. The Truth must be known to avoid the misery of birth and death." If we cradle this thought in our mind, it has the same effect as chanting, because what we think while eating will be emphasized. If we struggle to maintain ideal thought, however, chanting is prescribed. It is also best to remain silent while eating; if we speak, we should speak about a divine subject. Alternatively, we could listen to some devotional music that keeps our mind calm and quiet.

Just as meditation and worship are yajñas, sacrifices to please the deities, eating is also considered a yajña. How is this possible? The food we eat provides energy for our systems to cultivate divine qualities such as patience, endurance, calmness, quietness, and so on. A divine energy presides over each of these attributes and thereby resides in our bodies. We honor these deities by providing food that will enrich those good qualities. When we eat foods with the specific intention of honoring such qualities, we feed those deities and strengthen those qualities.

Each person needs different kinds of energy for various activities and at different times in life. A person acquires this energy through the food she eats. It is possible to direct our intention while eating so that the food provides us with the particular energy we need. The vehicle that delivers our intention to our digestive system is our *saliva*. It directs our digestive system to produce the energy that we need. The saliva of each person is unique and works according to one's intention. The mind directs the saliva, and the saliva directs the digestion according to the specific needs of each individual. This is the mechanism by which each person gains needed energy.

Like our thoughts and intentions, the emotions we feel as we are eating will be amplified. If we eat while we are experiencing overattachment to the external world, the overattachment will be reinforced. If we are egotistic or jealous while eating, those qualities will be strengthened. It is best to avoid eating while under the influence of such emotions. In contrast, if we are very humble at mealtimes, the food we eat will support our humility. This dynamic continues to operate until the food is digested.

POSTURES WHILE EATING

If we eat while we are walking or standing, we will be comparatively less stable than when sitting in a cross-legged posture. Our mind is more agitated when walking or standing, and it tends to be more fickle. Moreover, our food supports whatever activity we engage in while eating. If we are wandering from here to there while eating, our food will reinforce our capriciousness. It will support our unstable movements and external work rather than the internal movement that we desire. Furthermore, we will not properly digest our food.

This is the reason the āsana called *sukhāsana* is recommended for eating. Sukhāsana is a comfortable, stable posture in which we sit cross-legged on the floor. It promotes calmness and quietness. Eating while standing or sitting in a chair—while commonly practiced in the West—is not advisable. Standing will provoke a flow of both rajasic and tamasic energy in the body. Sitting in a chair, with the legs pointing downward, provokes a downward flow of tamasic energy. Thus, food consumed in these postures will tend to be converted to tamas and rajas energy. On the other hand, when sitting in sukhāsana, the legs will be folded and weight will be pressing against the feet. Therefore, the tamas energy, which moves from the navel to the feet, will be restricted. Moreover, this posture encourages an easy upward flow of energy that can provoke sattva in our system. Whatever we eat will be digested with this sattvic influence. This will help our meditation. For most Westerners this is an uncommon way of sitting and eating. It should be adopted as much as possible. If one's body is unable to sit in this way while eating, the use of supportive pillows or chairs is necessary.

For ten to fifteen minutes after eating, the digestive system works very strongly. Though it takes much longer overall, the main work is done soon after eating. That is why after eating, we should rest and maintain the same mindset as during the meal. We should not start serious work for a little while. Then our food will work according to our intention.

BATHING BEFORE MEALS

To promote success in our yogic practice, we need to convert the food that we eat into sattvic energy. This is possible only when the body and mind are already sattva dominant. External cleanliness and the touch of the water on our skin provoke sattva. Eating the right food after taking a bath further enhances sattva. This supports our whole system in becoming balanced. That is why it is best to eat only after taking a bath. However, if one takes an early morning bath, there is no need to repeat this before each meal.

If we are sleepy or tired and take a bath, we will feel refreshed and alert. If we have too much mental activity in our body, we feel calmer and more collected after a bath. These are all indications that taking a bath provokes sattvic energy. If we feel sleepy and tired, this points to tamasic energy in the body. A bath solves this problem. If we feel mentally agitated or jumpy, it indicates there is too much rajasic energy in the body. A bath may solve that problem, also.

When we sit for meditation, we want an abundance of sattvic energy in our system. Whenever we accumulate too much rajasic or tamasic energy, water is a wonderful cleanser. It works both internally and externally. We can cleanse our system of certain toxins by drinking water in a prescribed way as a discipline. We can cleanse the outside of our body by taking a bath, and in doing so promote sattvic energy.

Sometimes it is not possible to take a bath before eating. We may be traveling on a train or plane where no facilities are available. If it is not possible to take a bath, perhaps we could sit in a cool breeze, which also provokes sattva. While this is not as effective as taking a bath, it helps. Our mind will become quieter.

HANDLING FOOD

When we touch food with our hands, we can feel many of its characteristics, such as temperature and texture. We may not be able to identify all its characteristics, but knowingly or unknowingly, we gather a great deal of information about the food through touch. Our hands transmit energy from our body; they have the capacity to be powerful channels of sacred energy flow. This is why it is better to eat food with our hands than with utensils. Furthermore, it is better to eat food primarily with our right hand rather than with our left. This is because a beneficial energy for Realization flows through our right hand. When conveying a blessing, a sage will place his right palm on the recipient.

There is an astral channel, or nāḍī, in the palm of the right hand. If this nāḍī touches our food, the food will be made sacred. That touch even has the power to remove some of the impurities in food. In part, the palm indicates who a person is and what his intention is. When we touch food, the food changes to support our individual nature and intention. If we touch our food with a good intention, the impact of our touch further supports our main intention of Liberation.

Our body is composed of five basic elements: earth, water, fire, air, and space. We eat food to support these five basic elements, and our five fingers represent them. If we touch food with our five fingers, the elements in our body are better maintained by the food. A practitioner desires to develop his body to suit his internal path. Eating with the right hand promotes this intention.

Even if we eat with a spoon or a fork, we will still get some support for the five elements, because the food itself is the most important factor supporting these elements. Using utensils may not support our desire for Liberation to the maximum extent, however, because the food will build up our body in a way that is more suited for external activities.

TIMES FOR EATING

Our food affects us quite differently, depending on when we eat it. According to certain natural rhythms and cycles in the universe, there are specific times of the day when our digestive fire is activated more easily and readily. When our digestive fire is activated, it can easily convert sattvic food to sattvic energy throughout our system. If we provoke the digestive fire at other times, the food that we eat is converted into rajasic or tamasic energy. This is because our digestive fire does not function properly at other times of the day. It is not ready to function, but it is being forced to. We have provoked it at a time when it wants to be quiet.

In particular, food consumed at sunrise, sunset, or midnight will become rajasic or tamasic. This is because the system is not ready to digest food at these times. As a result, food will remain in the digestive tract for longer than normal. Unwanted reactions will occur in the food and it will cause us to become agitated and activated, or we will feel sleepy. Even though we may have eaten a sattvic dominant food, sattva will not be provoked. This is because our digestive system is not prepared to welcome these qualities. Instead, it will focus on the rajasic or tamasic qualities of that particular food. Based on one's individual constitution, one person may become more tamasic, while someone else may become more rajasic. In either case, we lose our meditative mood.

DIGESTIVE FIRE

Many people today suffer from what is considered "poor" or "weak" digestion. This is not simply a question of the *strength* of our digestion, however. The problem is that the nature of our digestion changes according to the natural rhythm and cycle of the body throughout the day.

Modern medicine sheds light on this, as well. Our digestive fire is a combination of many secretions, including pepsin, hydrochloric acid, bile, and other enzymes. Because there are variations of those secretions throughout the day, our digestion may be weak, or even not work at all, if we eat at the wrong times.

THREE ENERGIES AT WORK

The digestive fire also has its own nature, according to each individual. It can convert food into any of the three basic energy types, but this works according to an individual's constitution, saṃskāra, and intention. These three factors control the digestive fire. Of these factors, the influence of the constitution is the strongest—for the reason that we cannot change our constitution. The next strongest influence is saṃskāra, for we can never completely overcome the effects of our saṃskāra until final Liberation. After these two, our own intention has an impact on how we convert food into energy. Here we have the greatest measure of control over our digestive fire, because we can cultivate the intention to live a sattvic life. If we develop this intention to the maximum extent, then even if we have some rajasic and tamasic qualities, we will digest our food so that it will produce partially sattvic energy.

The proportion of sattvic, rajasic, and tamasic energies produced is based on the prominence of the three influencing factors. If a person is highly rajasic and at the same time has a sattvic intention, her food will produce more rajasic energy than sattvic. But that rajasic energy will be led by sattvic energy. This means that she will use his rajasic energy for sattvic purposes. Also, after the full use of his rajasic energy, she will feel an upwelling of sattva. She will be calmer and quieter. This is simply the grace of Nature. However, if a person is a fully sattvic person, and eats with a sattvic intention, the food will produce only sattvic energy.

Milk with sugar and cardamom is a very sattvic food. Both a yogi and a thief may consume such milk, according to their own intentions. The yogi has the intention to live a sattvic life. She will fully convert that milk into sattvic energy. Her mind will remain calm and sattvic. The thief has the intention to steal. He will convert that same drink into energy led by both his rajasic and tamasic intentions. In the end, he will steal something with that energy. Certainly, the milk will provide him with some sattvic energy, but he may use that energy to sit quietly and study his victims so that he may successfully make off with their possessions! The sattvic energy derived from the milk serves his rajasic intention.

If someone has a completely tamas-dominant constitution, and tamasic saṃskāras are working, it becomes inevitable that he will often eat at sunrise and sunset. A force from within will impel him to do so. Those are the times when he will be seriously interested in eating. His appetite will be strongest then; he will grab some food to eat and be highly satisfied. Because his system and constitution are tamasic, he needs some tamasic energy. This is the operating mechanism. So it may not be possible to change his food habits. If compelled to eat in a sattvic manner, he may rebel and find some other deviation that will supply the needed tamasic energy. He may alter what he eats, or he may increase his tamasic intention while eating. If he does not have enough tamasic energy in his system to fuel his tamasic activities, he will feel unhappy.

Just as eating at sunrise and sunset produces tamasic and rajasic energy, certain auspicious days throughout the year are meant for meditation. These days may be tracked by the Indian lunar calendar and the advice of a knowledgable yogi. They are particularly precious and are meant for yogic practice. We are given an opportunity to experience something deeper and more profound on those days than in our normal practice, and we are best served by taking advantage of it. The influence at those times is favorable for our yogic journey, so we need to avoid all other activities, including eating.

If we were to consume food at those times, the food would be converted into tamasic energy, and this would be a misuse of Nature's grace. Instead, if we sit quietly and do our meditation, we will be greatly benefited. Even if we are not aware of these auspicious days and times, Nature may indicate something to us directly. Every now and then, we may feel very quiet and happy spontaneously. When this happens, we can take advantage of it by forgoing eating any food and going somewhere to meditate.

EATING WITH OTHERS

As mentioned above, eating a meal in the company of others has an influence on us. If we eat with like-minded people who have the same energy as we do, their energy supports us and ours will support them. We share the same intention for eating food. We want to use food for Realization, and so do they. When many people with the same intention eat together, the digestion of each one will convert food to energy moving in the same direction.

Sometimes animals and birds will influence us. It will affect our food and digestion negatively if a salivating dog or other animal with an obvious craving for our meal watches us eat. If there is an animal watching us, we should feed the animal before we eat.

DRINKING WATER

Just as for eating food, there are disciplines for drinking water. We need to consume sufficient water at the appropriate times. When we are thirsty, we should drink water. If we do not drink enough water, our urine will be yellowish or reddish, rather than clear. Ideally, a person will pass urine six times per day. The frequency may vary sometimes. Those living in a dry area will pass urine less frequently than those in a humid area. Both need to drink sufficient water.

There is a misconception that drinking large quantities of water improves our health. Certainly, water purifies the system, but some foods purify our system, as well. Good food will absorb toxins and eliminate them. If we consume too much water, it causes two problems. First, it impedes the digestive process. Water does not need to be digested, but it provokes the system to secrete digestive juices. It also impairs our digestive capabilities by reducing heat in our system. Therefore, it is best not to consume a large amount of water immediately after a meal. The other problem with drinking too much water is water retention. While overconsumption of water is not the sole cause for water retention, it contributes to the problem.

Twenty-five percent of the stomach should be filled with water at each meal. In addition, we need to drink some water at other times of the day. One or two hours after each meal, we could drink some water. If we regularly drink water when we are not thirsty, we will gradually weaken our digestion.

The water that we drink with meals may be taken at different stages of the meal, depending on individual needs. Those who wish to lose weight should consume water before meals. Those who are very lean should drink water after meals. Those whose bodies are well proportioned should consume a little water after each dish to cleanse the tongue and palate. This discipline will also help the taste buds savor the food properly. The tongue and saliva dictate how food is digested. When we eat, it is best to experience the taste of our food to the maximum extent. When we fully taste the food, our digestive system will prepare itself to receive the food and will then work properly. Eating in a calm and quiet manner while tasting and enjoying each type of food has a beneficial impact on our body and mind.

Water cleanses the body, both inside and out. For this, yogic tradition recommends a practice called *uṣaḥpāna*. Uṣaḥpana is the practice of drinking eight cupped handfuls of water early in the morning shortly after morning meditation. If we hold our hands together to form a cup, we can measure a certain quantity of water that will suit each of us based on our size. A small person will hold less water than a large person; thus, a small person will drink less than a large person in this practice. This practice should be done prior to sunrise, on an empty stomach, and after brushing the teeth. The water will work through the system within one to two hours, causing urination once or twice within that period. Clear urine indicates that the system has been cleaned and flushed. The urination that accompanies this practice is in addition to the usual six times per day.

This practice is not for quenching thirst. It is only for purification. There are many benefits to this practice. If we practice uṣaḥpana regularly, our appetite will be stimulated at the right time. Uṣaḥpana eliminates impurities and promotes regular and healthy movement of the bowels. As a result of the practice of uṣaḥpana, we will feel a lightness and freshness in the body. We will feel less drowsiness.

If we draw the water at night and keep it in a copper vessel until morning, the copper will have a mild laxative effect on our system.

Over time, the copper vessel will oxidize, so it should be cleaned with lemon or tamarind juice mixed with ash and a little bit of mud. Chlorinated water will react with the copper and disturb one's health, so it is better to use purified water. If this is not possible, one can boil the water at night before putting it in the copper vessel, and the chlorine will evaporate, though boiling the water will cause it to lose certain other properties, as well.

These days, it is difficult to find pure, natural water. Distilled water is not optimal for health. Although it is pure, it is missing some necessary minerals. In an area that is unpolluted, rainwater is the best water to drink. After the rain starts, wait a few minutes and then collect it. The dust will settle in those first few minutes, and the remaining rainwater will be pure. However, today heavy pollution is widespread, and toxins like sulfuric acid and even radiation can be carried great distances in rain clouds. Ingesting such water is totally contrary to good health and should be avoided.

Some sādhus and yoga practitioners in India live near lakes and streams. Many practice the discipline of using only natural water. Daily, they carry pots and jugs to the water's edge and collect it. Some will not use water that comes from a pipe or a bore well under any circumstances. These practitioners are following a piece of yogic advice to drink only water that has been exposed to the sun and air. They feel that water collected in this way will be much better than water that comes from a well or through a pipe. They also appreciate water collected near where precious herbs grow on the bank of a river or stream.

SALIVA

Each person has her own fate. She has her own constitution and needs to consume food that will provide the energy required for her constitution. She will digest her food in a way that is unique to her. For these reasons, yogis recommend certain disciplines regarding one's saliva. Saliva plays an enormous role in our individual digestive processes. This is poorly understood today. Saliva is an energy that works in harmony with many other aspects of our system. It contains unique properties linked to the mind of each individual. Transmission of saliva between different individuals—for example, when sharing plates and utensils—has the propensity to cause imbalance in one's digestion, and even may provoke mental disturbances.

Saliva may be unintentionally shared between individuals either directly or indirectly. If someone has eaten from a spoon or fork and then touches that utensil to our plate, this is a direct sharing, or connection. If we eat food from which someone else has taken a bite, this is a direct connection, as well. This direct sharing, or connection between individuals, has the strongest negative impact on us.

The connection may also be indirect. Saliva is energy. If someone has eaten food in a certain place, and we sit in that place to eat, the energy from the other person's saliva will affect us. Therefore, it is better to wash a spot with a little water before eating in the same location where someone else has previously eaten. If the sun shines on that spot for a short period of time, that can also reduce the energetic impact of another person. The awareness of these influencing factors should not lead to fear, judgment, or prejudice against others. Rather, it is honoring our differences and respecting what is needed to maintain a balanced system. Just as we should take care to limit the influence of others' energies on us, we must take care to limit our own influences on others.

Because of the strong impact saliva carries, certain disciplines are recommended while cooking and serving. First, if we taste food while preparing it and then put the cooking spoon back in the pot, this will have a negative effect on all those who eat the meal. Instead of providing a service to them by cooking, we will have done them a disservice.

When serving food, the best practice is to have one person serve food to all others who are eating. This way, the server can keep his hands clean. If someone who is eating must also serve more food, that person should wash his hands before touching the serving utensil or the pot of food. When placing food on a plate from which someone has already eaten, the serving utensil should not touch the plate. Instead, the food should be dropped from just above the plate; it may take a bit of practice to do this without splashing food.

There are two exceptions to this discipline. A couple who shares a deeply devoted love will not be harmed by sharing saliva during the deep expression of their love. In addition, touching the saliva of a baby or child under the age of five will not disturb us. Yogic philosophy says that a baby is very near to the Eternal Truth. This is before the saṃskāra of that baby begins operating fully. When serving food to the baby, we need not be concerned about coming into contact with her saliva.

INDIRECT EFFECTS ON FOOD

The quality of our food can be affected indirectly by how we earn money to purchase that food. As we mentioned in our discussion on ahimsā, or nonviolence, if we earn our money for food through violence, then even if it is inherently sattvic food, such as rice or milk, it will carry rajasic and tamasic qualities. The proportion of sattvic, rajasic, and tamasic qualities will vary based on the nature of the violence. If the violence was strong, the influence will be highly tamasic. If the violence was weak, the food will retain its sattvic quality, with a small tamasic influence. All food that comes from a violent or dishonest deed causes a blockage on the yogic path. Alternatively, if we buy sattvic food with money that we earned in a sattvic manner, the food will be very sattvic.

In general, a very healthy person will have an honorable source of income. However, sometimes a person may seem to be quite healthy and happy, even though he is doing something wrong or is engaged in dishonorable work. This is due to some other good karma that is working in the present. But behind the veil of ignorance, corrective karma based on those current misdeeds is waiting to unfold. A common person cannot see this, but yogis can.

Moreover, sometimes we are not able to understand the nature of proper health, and so we will be easily misled. We see a person who looks healthy and totally happy, but her problems are only hidden from view. Already she may be experiencing the results of gaining money improperly, and these results may already be exerting an intense and even unbearable pressure on her. If such a person practices yoga, she will not have positive results. From one side, she may be making great effort, doing many practices; from another side, she is gaining her livelihood in a way that causes acute suffering to others. The influence of money acquired in this fashion will be stronger than the spiritual effort that she is putting forth. Finally, she will be disappointed, declare that yogic practices are invalid, and eventually renounce them. If she is a truly lucky yoga practitioner, she will lose all of the assets that she gained through violence. She may feel cursed by Nature, but in reality she has received the grace of God. Thereafter, she may have some degree of anxiety because of her loss, but this is simply a karmic remnant. Overall, she will find that her yoga practice has vastly improved.

WHAT IS FOOD?

Let us ask ourselves again, What really is food? We are given many different kinds of nourishment for the health and growth of our body and mind. As we saw in our discussion of mitāhāra, *anything* we receive from the external universe is food. This means that food is not only what we ingest with our mouths but also includes the air we breathe, light, sound—and even knowledge. All of this is āhāra—food—in one sense.

Light. The light that illuminates this world is considered āhāra. Previously, people lived very naturally, and their use of light was primarily limited to the daylight hours. They might have used a candle or oil lamp in the evening, but such sources of light are small and relatively harmless.

Today, with electric lights, we have the capacity to use light excessively, which causes much disturbance to the body and mind. The early night hours are meant for relaxing, light entertainment, and eating a little food. The later night hours are meant for sleep. Night hours are not meant for hard work, deep thinking, or stimulating entertainment. The problem is that electric lights have reduced our relaxation and sleep. They provoke thoughts and hard work, and they strain the eyes. The eyes need relaxation just like all other organs; our use of electric lights has greatly compromised the opportunity for the eyes to relax.

If we go to bed late at night, and then sleep late, we may feel that we have received sufficient rest. But yoga contends that our sleep will not be ultimately relaxing. The night is meant for sleeping. Then alone is full relaxation possible.

The hours for sleep are from approximately 9 P.M. to 4 A.M. (corresponding to a 6 P.M. sunset and 6 A.M. sunrise). If we want to go to sleep at 9 P.M., we must eat some light food at 7:30 or 8 P.M., and then prepare for sleep. This preparation does not include bright lights and busy work. If we engage in hectic activity up until 9 P.M., we will not be ready to sleep for another hour or two after that. Bright lights and TV in the evening are disturbing to the cycles of the body.

Air. Air is also āhāra. Today, because of our busy lifestyle, our breathing is disturbed. We do not exhale and inhale properly. Many will not inhale and exhale fully because of stress and strain in their busy daily lives. This stress needs to be fully eliminated. If we visit small villages, where the inhabitants live quite naturally, we will see a difference in their style of breathing due to the calm and quiet environment. We need to slow down and live quieter lives; otherwise, our yoga practice will not yield the best possible results. Only then will our breathing have a chance to correct itself.

There are other problems associated with air and breathing. Sometimes we live where there is no proper ventilation, or, conversely, in a place that is overventilated. Neither helps our yoga practice. Ideally, there should be some cross-ventilation but not too much. If wind is constantly blowing through the house, excessive vāta will be provoked; those who live in such a house will have breathing disturbances caused by too much vāta. But in today's cities, often there is too little ventilation. In this case, the air will become stale and polluted. We will inhale too many toxins and not enough fresh air.

An ideal house will be open, unencumbered by restrictions on its sides, such as other buildings or high walls. Instead, some beneficial plants, trees, and herbs will grow on all sides. These will partially block the wind and add a calming quality to the air. We will feel healthier because the air is fresh. This is what is ideal for a yoga practitioner. Unfortunately, today it is difficult to find these things. These are all problems related to mitāhāra.

Media. Food is everything that we experience in this universe through our five senses. We receive information from various media like television, books, radio, and the Internet; we also attend lectures, watch films, and take walks in nature. In one way or another, all of these activities are food for our minds and hearts. These foods have tremendous influence on our systems. Our entire life may be influenced by these forms of āhāra.

Just as the food we eat through our mouths can cause great disturbances in our minds and bodies, so too these types of media foods can cause disturbances in our systems. For instance, young children who are exposed to sex through the media may develop early sexual maturity. Such influences may affect one's whole life and lead to great tragedy. Some media, including music, that are considered "entertainment" may have a powerfully negative impact on our mind. In order to cultivate a calm and quiet life, we should be very careful and discriminate in choosing what we "eat" in this sense.

The above disciplines associated with mitāhāra are recommended primarily for one who is doing an intense practice. Such a person wants to reach the final goal as soon as possible, and thus uses every available method. However, once one has achieved Realization, one may practice fewer food disciplines than before. A Realized person will have developed the capacity to overcome the ill effects that would hurt a common person. Once a person has reached the final goal, there is no need to follow all the disciplines, but one may still decide to do so in order to set an example, and to encourage others to live more meaningful lives.

PRECIOUS FOOD

Under certain conditions, food is considered precious: when it has been purchased with money acquired in an honorable fashion; when it has been prepared from sattvic ingredients by a cook with a yogic mentality; when it has been prepared into delicious dishes that satisfy our taste; and when it is consumed in the correct quantity, at the right time, and with the best intentions. Those who consume precious food and develop the resulting sense of balance in their lives soon find little satisfaction with anything less. If a practitioner consumes precious food for twelve years or more, there will be a radical shift and restructuring in her body. It paves the way for Realization and Liberation.

If we regularly consume precious food, our meditation will be easier. For many who do not eat precious food, meditation will be a form of torture. They will fail in their efforts. They make time for their practice; they sit every morning and evening; they read spiritual books and hear the words of Realized teachers; but their body and mind will not co-operate because of their food practices. They may struggle for a long time until they finally realize their efforts are being wasted. By becoming firmly established in the principles of mitāhāra, we will tame our body and mind, experience less disturbance, and our yogic practice will yield better results.

Nature has endowed all human beings and creatures on this planet with a body, and the universe provides food for all beings with bodies. Nature's purpose in supplying everyone with food is for the enjoyment of Realization and Liberation.

The human body is the most wondrous of all bodies in the world. It is given to us by the grace of Nature. Through it, we are meant to enjoy wonderful yogic experiences. We need to nurture and maintain our bodies through food. Nature has provided us with this body, so Nature also will provide food for it.

In India, another short prayer recited before eating is "Oh, goddess Annapūrṇā, you are all pervading. You are the escort of Śiva. I beg alms from you with an intention to realize Truth and to become detached. Please offer me alms." Only after we say one or more of these prayers will we eat the food.

CONCLUSION

These sections describing the yamas offer only preliminary advice for the journey toward Realization. Unless these disciplines and preparations are either inherent or developed fully, our journey will be less successful. Though some of these disciplines seem like minor issues when compared to the final goal, their importance cannot be overstated. Unless our problems with this external world can be solved or eliminated, we will not be capable of moving to the internal world.

As we have tried to show, each of the yamas is its own path to Realization and Liberation. When we follow any yama to its depth, it automatically brings all other yamas (and niyamas, discussed in chapter 8) into alignment. Each yama links with the other yamas like the threads of a spider's web. When we show mercy toward others, we will not hurt them; when we are tolerant and steadfast in our behavior, we will be resilient to the inevitable changes in our lives.

An aspirant may feel that certain yogic techniques are more important than these disciplines. He may think that prāṇāyāma can control the mind and that nothing more is needed for Realization. He may think that meditation alone is the key to Samādhi. Or he may believe that when these yogic techniques are mastered, other disciplines relating to ethical behavior and healthy living are of comparatively little importance.

These attitudes demonstrate a profound lack of understanding about the nature of Realization and Liberation. They also reflect a deep misunderstanding about the importance of preparing the body and mind to be supportive vehicles to reach these noble destinations. Though the yamas pertain to the external world, they are essential for an aspirant to move internally. Without them, a person might practice for years and end up no closer to the target than when they began.

CHAPTER EIGHT

THE NIYAMAS

इन्द्रियनिग्रहः

BECAUSE WE HAVE LOST our original connection with the Eternal Truth, the yogic journey requires perseverance and dedication. Our primary effort must be to bring balance, realignment, and harmony to the body, mind, and senses. The path of Aṣṭāṅga Yoga helps us develop the necessary practices to realign our system and correct the imbalances that we have developed over many lifetimes. These corrective measures happen in two ways: *externally* and *internally*.

External alignment involves telling the truth, practicing nonviolence, paying attention to our food, and all the other yamas we have previously explained. The yamas focus on these external disciplines with the purpose of changing our behavior in the external world.

The *niyamas* focus mostly on *internal* disciplines and practices, and deal largely with the mind. This includes cultivating contentment, study of the Self, and surrendering to the Eternal Truth.

The word *yama* means "discipline" or "control." The words *yama* and *niyama* have almost identical meanings except that *ni* means "intense." The internal practices are often considered more rigorous and difficult than the external ones. However, the external effort of the yamas prepares the mind for the internal effort of the niyamas. Initially, we may find it easier to change some of our external behaviors; after we gain a measure of control externally, we may find it easier to focus on internal disciplines. Also, in the beginning, internal problems may be more difficult to identify, let alone correct. Therefore, we should clear the external problems as much as possible. During that process, we will develop the skill and confidence necessary to take a more internal approach to our practice. While there is thus some natural progression, these two limbs do need to happen simultaneously in order to make significant changes in our system.

According to Patañjali, there are five niyamas: *śauca, santoṣa, tapas, svādhyāya,* and *Īśvara praṇidhāna.* These translate as *cleanliness, contentment, austerity* or *penance, study of the Self,* and *surrender to the Eternal Truth.*

As with the yamas, the sage Yājñavalkya lists ten niyamas, which vary slightly from Patañjali's five. Yājñavalkya's niyamas additionally include *āstikya* as faith in the Eternal Truth or God; *dāna* as spiritual offering; *hrīhi* as a type of humility; *mati* as decisiveness; *japa* as chanting; and *vrata* as a kind of self-discipline. Yājñavalkya also speaks of Īśvara *pūjana,* which refers to the worship of Īśvara, or God, and is similar to Patañjali's description of Īśvara praṇidhāna. In the same way, Yājñavalkya's description of *siddhānta śravaṇa* is similar to Patañjali's explanation of *svādhyāya.* Like Patañjali, Yājñavalkya defines *santoṣa* as contentment but includes it in his discussion of the yamas. For this book's purpose, we will discuss twelve niyamas: śauca, santoṣa, tapas, svādhyāya, Īśvara praṇidhāna, āstikya, dāna, hrīhi, mati, japa, vrata, and siddhānta śravaṇa.

ŚAUCA: PHYSICAL CLEANLINESS

The yogi's mind should be sattva dominant and always ready to move in an upward direction. For this reason, the mind itself is sometimes referred to as *sattva.* In order to maintain this sattvic domination, one must try to avoid contact with obstructive influences. This is primarily why śauca, or cleanliness, holds such importance in yoga teachings.

There are two types of cleanliness: *physical* and *mental.* The condition we experience after perspiring is an example of being physically *unclean.* We generally seek to bathe away these toxins from the surface of our bodies. Examples of mental *uncleanliness* are unsuitable desire, anger, greed, ignorance, egotism, and jealousy. Once we begin to calm and quiet our mind, we will easily notice the effect these physical and mental experiences have on our meditation. As we pay closer attention, we see a relationship between physical and mental cleanliness.

TWO TYPES OF PHYSICAL CLEANLINESS

There are two distinct approaches to physical cleanliness. The first approach involves the removal of toxins and impurities from the body. Some of these toxins are produced inside the body and make their way to the surface; others attach to the surface of the body from the external environment. The second approach of śauca is to avoid bodily contact with certain *materials, places, animals, plants,* and *other human beings* that disturb our mind.

We can eliminate many types of impurities by simply washing our body. Most of the body is made up of water and earth elements. If we use water and an earth element like clay to clean our external body, we establish a link between our body and the earth. In India, there is a practice of mixing very fine-grained clay with water to be used for cleansing the body. The mixture is smooth and soft but abrasive enough to exfoliate impurities and toxins. In many parts of the world, mudpacks, facials, and cleansers contain clay as an essential ingredient.

ELIMINATION

There are also disciplines of śauca associated with the elimination of waste through urination and bowel movements. When we touch certain external substances, they transmit impurities that disturb the mind. Perhaps the most obvious example is human feces, which has a strong negative impact on the mind and body. Even though excrement is part of our body before we eliminate it, its reaction with the external world makes it very toxic to our systems. Contact with another person's excrement has an even greater negative impact. If by chance we touch feces, it is our duty, at the very least, to wash our hands and feet as soon as possible. The water counteracts the negative influence and helps to reduce its adverse effects.

This brings up the question of how to cleanse oneself after having a bowel movement. Although most Westerners use toilet paper, many people around the world prefer to clean themselves with water. Washing with water is very effective in removing many negative influences on the body.

When we feel the urge for elimination, various effects occur in the body. First, there is a slight secretion in the mouth. In addition, a slight external heat is generated on the surface of the eyes and the feet. If one pays close attention while on the toilet, one can easily notice these things. These all have a slight disturbing effect on the mind during meditation practice.

To counteract their effect, we should rinse our mouth with a little bit of water immediately after using the toilet. This should be repeated three or four times. We should also wash our hands and feet, as well as put a little water on the eyelids to cool them. These cleansing disciplines will help our mind become calm and quiet.

A short, cool bath in a river or lake is recommended before morning and evening yoga practice as a way to help calm the mind and enable us to sit quietly. When a natural source of water is unavailable, one may take a cool shower or bucket bath. A healthy person will have a bowel movement in the early morning and early evening. This simplifies the sequence of bathing and practicing. Unfortunately, many of us find that our bodies are not in harmony with this ideal schedule, and our bowel movements are irregular. Also, in certain situations, it may be impossible to bathe prior to practicing. When the circumstances are not ideal, we do the best we can and may simply wash our hands, face, and feet. Most important, we should hold the ideal in our mind.

INFLUENCE OF TOUCH

Sometimes physical contact with certain animals, plants, and even other human beings can be disturbing to our yoga practice. This is an issue when the dominant energy in their systems strongly clashes with our own.

For example, much to the dismay of many Westerners, yoga discourages the touch of dogs and cats because such touch is detrimental to yogic practice. For example, dogs have an acute connection to their senses and are very rajasic by nature. They should be very active and attached to their senses—it is their nature to wake easily throughout the night in response to sounds or smells and to go investigate. Dogs are praised for remaining alert to their environment and guarding their owners. This excess of activity is natural for them.

However, touching a dog transfers these rajasic qualities to us. The touch of the dog will provoke many thoughts and a tendency toward extroverted behavior. We may even develop a greater sensitivity to hearing and smell. If we frequently come into contact with dogs, we will lose our ability to utilize the sattvic energy that prevails at sunrise and sunset. In due course, this will hamper our sleep and our yoga practice.

In the West, many people have deep emotional connections to dogs and cats. Once we have adopted them as pets, it is difficult to send them away. These animals may even have some positive influence for people who otherwise feel isolated. It is also possible that, because dogs and cats in the Western world are less wild than in India, they may be slightly less rajasic by nature; therefore, their influence may not be as detrimental. At the same time, serious yoga practitioners may still feel some negative influence from their pets, so it is advisable for pet owners to bathe before practicing yoga. If that is not possible, they should simply wash the hands, feet, and face.

The touch of lizards, snakes, and other reptiles also disturb the mind for yoga practice. It is better not to keep these animals as pets. Touching donkeys, pigs, eagles, and crows is considered inauspicious, as well. On the other hand, touching a sparrow, parrot, deer, cow, horse, elephant, peacock, or swan tends to have a quieting effect on the mind.

A serious practitioner will feel the influence of another person's touch on his meditation. The touch of some human beings can have a powerfully negative effect on one's practice. If one comes into physical contact with such a person, it can have both direct and indirect influences. No one fully knows the condition of another's mind, nor does one know whether that person is calm and kind-hearted, greedy, cruel, or overly sexual. The more one touches others, the more one's mind will be influenced by that physical contact. It may simply prevent one from sitting quietly, or it may even provoke thoughts that lead one to emulate another person's dysfunctional behavior. For this reason, yogis recommend that one touch strangers as little as possible.

There are stories about a contemporary yogi who allowed certain people near him but strongly reacted to the physical proximity of others. Although it seemed like this yogi displayed preferential treatment, that was not true. The truth was that some people had energy that clashed with his energy: When he felt that variance, an aversion was activated within him, and he would simply ward off the conflicting energy.

Some people will not touch certain types of physical materials and yet are drawn to touch other types of materials. Often, their aversion and attraction are completely unconscious. We see this dynamic throughout all humankind. This is a demonstration of the principle of aversion and attraction of energy. We witness this same automatic and unconscious behavior in some varieties of animals and birds that avoid energy clashes very carefully. Sometimes an animal carefully avoids another type of animal, even though the other animal offers no threat. In other cases, animals find a peculiar type of attraction to another species. For example, some birds ride on the backs of buffalo to eat insects. There is a particular attraction between their energies, quite apart from the obvious benefits each provides the other.

In the West, the social customs include shaking hands and hugging. If we do not follow these customs, we may hurt others' feelings or cause misunderstandings. In such cases, sometimes it is better to simply follow the customs of the society and exercise common sense. If we feel that we have touched too many people, or that we have touched someone who carried some negative influence, we can take a bath before our yoga practice. A bath will solve many of the problems caused by touching rajasic or tamasic animals and people.

BENEFICIAL TOUCH

Not all touch is harmful to us. When we love someone deeply, his or her touch will not disturb our practice, providing the touch is mutually agreeable, timely, and meaningful. In the same way, we may wish to touch someone toward whom we feel great honor. An example of this is seen in India when an aspirant salutes his teacher or another honorable elder by touching his feet. However, in such a case, we should receive permission first.

As discussed previously, the touch of a baby is not disturbing and may even bring a calmness and quietness to our mind. At the same time, we must be careful that our touch does not adversely affect the baby. Not everyone's energy will be compatible with a baby's energy.

There are ways that we can recognize some of the signs of incompatibility. For example, the baby might start crying or seem disturbed after the touch of someone unfamiliar. Or the baby's skin color may become pale within a couple of days. This is one reason yoga suggests that we should not allow strangers to touch young babies. In India, pregnant women will conceal their bellies from the eyes of strangers. Like touching, looking also carries energy from one person to another and is therefore a form of touching. This understanding has been honored in India for ages.

At the same time, the touch of a Realized person will have a very favorable influence upon us. For this reason it is honored by yoga practitioners. In particular, touching the feet of a Realized teacher is considered powerful and beneficial. However, as mentioned above, such a touch is given with the permission of and at the discretion of the teacher.

NEGATIVE INFLUENCES OF TOUCH

We should not touch the family members of a Soul that has just entered or left a body. In other words, we should not touch members of families who have just experienced birth or death. These two periods of time are called *aśauca* in Saṃskṛta.

In India during these times, families follow certain disciplines, which include avoiding touching others. Many societies observe similar practices. The sadness of the Soul experiencing death has a strong influence on the Soul's relatives. At the time of death, the Soul that was living in the body loses everything related to the material world. In most cases, the Soul is forcibly dragged away from this world—from its loved ones, its home, its money, and all its earthly possessions. The sense of loss causes a great deal of pain. As a tree suffers when a branch is cut, so, too, a family suffers when a member of that family is lost.

Whether consciously felt or not, this sadness will linger for a certain period in the form of tamasic energy. If members of the grieving family touch other people, their touch transmits this tamasic energy to those they touch. This tamasic energy will then disturb other people's mental conditions and meditations.

We know that sadness loses its potency over time. This is common for all human beings. However, the grieving period varies from individual to individual. Some people become highly attached. When someone dies, they cry, wail, and throw themselves on the body of the deceased. For these people, the impact of the death will remain for a longer period of time. For them, the sanction against touching may last for thirty or forty days.

People who have a different perspective on life may feel sad when a loved one dies but not excessively sad. These people understand that death is common to all. Even when a close relative dies, such people know that they must adjust, and they may do so without intense grieving. For them, death is simply one more thing to accept. Since death comes to all, it is not something they view as extraordinary. They may return to a normal state of mind after only a few days, and the sanction against touching them may be shorter.

In India, the specific number of days one observes aśauca is linked to one's caste and lasts no longer than forty days. After the period of restriction is over, the family washes all their clothes, bathes, and then resumes normal interactions with other people. At that point, there are no further negative ramifications if they touch others.

In traditional teachings, it was believed that menstruating women should avoid touching and being touched. There is a short, three-day period when their systems are highly influenced by rajasic energy, as well as a downward movement of tamasic energy. These energies are thought to have the power to disturb other people's meditation practice and inner journey for an extended period of time. If touch occured during this period, people could minimize its influence simply by bathing. Though some Westerners find these teachings difficult to accept, they should be viewed through a traditional lens, and respected and honored because of the serious effect this type of touch has on one's practice.

Yoga and Modern Science

Modern science may not accept many of the ideas of yogic philosophy, but there are also many gaps in the knowledge of modern science. Scientists understand a tremendous amount about atoms, protons, electrons, and neutrons. They have developed theories about quarks, relativity, and quantum mechanics. But even with all of this knowledge, the two primary theories modern science uses to explain the universe—the theory of relativity and the theory supporting quantum mechanics—are diametrically opposed to each other!

Modern science does not acknowledge the reality of Samādhi, the highest state of human experience; nor does it accept the existence of prāṇa, the life force throughout the universe. When scientists do not understand something, they often dismiss it as mythical, unscientific, imaginary, or superstitious. Yet, the biggest problem is that they have not been able to properly *measure* the results or effects of these phenomena. And this is largely due to the limited scientific attention given to these phenomena. In the future, modern science may be able to measure and verify many of these things, including the consequences of touching. There are still great possibilities for discovery in these areas.

Nevertheless, strict yoga practitioners will adhere to these practices closely. Many Realized individuals, such as Ramakrishna Paramahamsa and Ramana Maharshi, followed many of these practices. However, we need not accept these ideas on faith alone; rather, we should test and validate them for ourselves. This requires a capacity to keenly observe subtle changes. The next time you happen to have close contact with someone related to a newborn baby, recently bereaved, or menstruating, simply observe your next meditation practice. Just as a small leaf can easily disturb the surface of a quiet lake, a calm and quiet mind will easily assess the difference. On the other hand, if the lake is already disturbed by buffalo and elephants, then even a large stone thrown into the water will hardly be noticed.

CLOTHING

According to the observation of yogis, the type of clothing we wear is very important because the properties of the fabric have an effect on us. For example, cotton is a good choice for clothing. Though it absorbs the energy of another's touch relatively easily, washing it removes all energetic influences. Hence, it is wise to launder cotton clothing between uses. Silk is more difficult to maintain, but it shields our system from impurities much better than other materials. When we wear silk, we can even sit in a place where many others have previously sat and not experience much transference of energy.

On the other hand, plastic and synthetic materials can be very disturbing to our body and should be avoided if possible. Today these materials appear everywhere, however, and often cannot be easily avoided. Nonetheless we should try to avoid direct contact if possible and minimize these articles in our wardrobe. This is because yogis have recently ascertained that plastic and synthetic articles block the flow of our body's energy. Moreover, plastic and synthetic materials have their own energy that is not harmonious with our own.

Today, many people own household items or clothing made from leather or other animal skins. In general, we should avoid touching animal skins because they influence us adversely. We should bathe after we touch them. There are some exceptions to this rule: animal skins such as those of the deer, cow, and tiger may have beneficial qualities, depending upon how the animal died and how their skins were acquired.

FOOD

Like the things we touch, the food we eat leaves an enormous impact on our practice. The ramifications of food having a negative influence will be much greater than even touching. This is because food goes into our bloodstream and remains there until the body can purge it, and this is not always easily accomplished.

When an aspirant has consumed non-ideal food over a long period of time, yogis recommend various types of fasting (described later in the third niyama, tapas). Fasting burns up any toxins stored in the bloodstream. Though fasting may be difficult for some people, it will eliminate most problems, and an aspirant will feel much better afterward.

HOUSEHOLD CLEANING

There are other practices we need to be aware of in terms of cleanliness. In preparation for yoga practice, it is best to avoid touching our shoes. Various unclean substances are found on the ground, and shoes easily pick up their influences. Similarly, it is better to avoid touching common household cleaning equipment like brooms, dusters, vacuum cleaners, and so on. These items come into contact with many unclean surfaces and carry disturbing influences. In traditional Indian houses, one will sweep and clean the house immediately before taking the daily bath. This allows a householder to complete his work and then remove the unwanted influences before his yoga practice.

LARGER IMPLICATIONS OF CLEANLINESS

Patañjali has pointed out other benefits of keeping our system clean. As we repeatedly clean our body, we begin to notice that we are regularly washing away impurities that come from inside. We begin to understand that the reason the physical body constantly secretes and excretes toxins is that it is not very pure. There are many impurities that the body has consumed through food, air, water, touch, and so on. This should not lead a practitioner to develop compulsive behaviors around cleanliness, nor should this lead to a fear of germs and contamination. By maintaining our clear intention, we may lose a level of egotism and attachment related to this body. Our egotism will be replaced with a deep understanding that this body is simply a tool or vehicle that takes us to our destination. At the same time, it is our duty to keep it well maintained, so that it can serve us in the optimal way. This attitude strengthens detachment. We may also arrive at this conclusion unconsciously, simply by keeping our body clean.

Moreover, by observing the constant degradation and destruction of the body, we gain a deeper understanding of its impermanence. Our body is not a house built on a rock; it is a house built on sand. When we maintain the principles of cleanliness, we become established in this knowledge. We gradually gain profound understanding about the fundamental nature of the body. This understanding will benefit us on our yogic journey.

CONTACT WITH OTHERS' BODIES

The various principles of śauca, which teach us about our own body, also provide an opportunity to better understand the bodies of others. Gradually, practitioners come to understand that as their own body is neither pure nor eternal, neither is anyone else's. While we may hesitate to touch other people as freely as we once did, we may come to develop more love for their Souls. This further reduces body-oriented attachments. It can also mitigate misunderstandings and complications that arise from touching others too freely. Our insights will help balance our systems and prepare us for our yogic practice. Even though there are many undesirable aspects related to the body, it is the most wonderful tool for crossing this ocean of birth and death. We must simultaneously value this body and accept its limitations.

MENTAL CLEANLINESS

Just as a wonderful fruit-yielding tree can be attacked by worms and insects, so, too, the mind can be attacked by impurities and destructive mental enemies. There are six such enemies that take shelter in the mind, known altogether as *ariṣaḍvarga.* They are primarily caused by unsuitable desires, and one must always be mindful of their mischievous nature.

These six enemies are *kāma,* unsuitable desire; *krodha,* untimely anger; *lobha,* unwise greed; *moha,* unfavorable ignorance; *mada,* unfavorable egotism; and *mātsarya,* unhealthy jealousy. These are the main enemies that live in one's mind and can easily spoil one's path. Using the power of māyā, they possess an uncanny ability to appear one moment and hide the next. Their nature is described by the word *kāmarūpi,* or "that which has the ability to change form." This is explained in ancient legends about demons that appear before a devotee in the form of an honored god or goddess in order to deceive and trick the devotee.

Only a few individuals on the yogic path will have *direct* experience of divine spheres. Most practitioners will experience these *un*-divine energies in the form of ignoble and dishonorable qualities. However, true to their deceptive nature, they will hide behind the mask of noble qualities. In this way, their deceit and trickery are quite ingenious and remarkable. They use all these tricks and devices to attack an individual and avoid detection.

These un-divine energies are in perpetual conflict with divine energies. Our body is their battlefield. When divine energies succeed, there is peace, happiness, contentment, Realization, and Liberation. When ignoble energies dominate, there is suffering, bondage, and rebirth.

This is why we should try to cultivate noble qualities through all means. We achieve such qualities through external practice of the yamas, such as nonviolence, truthfulness, eating sattvic food, and so on. We must also follow the internal disciplines of the niyamas, such as cleanliness, contentment, faith, and so on.

My great Eternal Teacher, Śrī Raṅga, cautioned, "Do not fight against these ignoble, demeaning energies. You cannot win. Just when you think you've overcome one, it will deceive you by wearing a mask of a noble quality. So do not bother about them. Focus instead on strengthening your noble qualities. These will fight on your behalf. You only need to be a witness. Day by day the ignoble qualities will begin to vanish once they discover there is no room for them at your home—your mind!"

Yoga is nothing but nurturing noble energy through all possible means. When these energies are denied food and shelter, they will lose their power and effectiveness. Eventually, they will vanish. This is the ultimate goal. Short of this, one should listen to and study the great yogic narrated stories such as the Rāmāyaṇa and the Mahābhārata. These possess a treasure house of knowledge to rid us of our ignorance and attachments. They contain a source of information about the grandeur of the Divine. Simply by hearing these stories, one can develop confidence and understanding. Gradually, one will be led to develop a more and more ideal way of life.

PROVOKING SATTVA

Nature can provoke sattva much more easily when we follow the principles of cleanliness. While sattvic energy manifests in everyone's body, it comes at a particular time and by a specific method for each individual. If we are relatively free from the influence of others, the cycle of sattva works correctly. If we are heavily influenced by others, the sattvic cycle becomes hindered. Patañjali wrote about sattva *śuddhi,* which means "purity of sattva." We gain sattva śuddhi when we practice the principles of cleanliness. Our bodies naturally have plenty of sattvic energy available to them. If we simultaneously eliminate impurities and toxins while practicing cleanliness, sattva will begin to dominate. When we experience this pure sattva in our system, we can use it for our yogic practice.

Abundant sattvic energy in the system leads to detachment. Through appropriate detachment, we develop a clear mind and correct mentality. However, one who is lacking sattva domination will be constantly disturbed. Because of this disturbance, mental tendencies such as violence, greed, and jealousy develop. An enlightened mentality emerges through a relaxed mind. That relaxation is possible only with the provocation of pure sattva. When we cannot relax, our thoughts may become negative and unmanageable. We may lose our good-heartedness and other favorable qualities of mind. For these reasons, each of us should regularly have periods of pure sattva provocation and relaxation.

One who is very good-hearted gradually develops a capacity for single-focused concentration, or *ekāgratā* in Saṃskṛta. Ekāgratā is essential for yoga practice. Meditation, the gateway to Samādhi, requires the ability to focus on one object. Each practitioner needs to acquire this ability. Both total relaxation and the ability to focus rely on practicing the principles of cleanliness, or śauca.

There are a very few people who, since birth, possess a supreme level of concentration and do not need to practice these disciplines. Most of us do best to follow these disciplines, unless advised otherwise by a yogi. Furthermore, those of us who develop more and more one-pointedness will be able to overcome the distractions from the five senses. As we sit for meditation, our senses will try to drag our mind to the external world. The only reason our senses have the power to do that is that the mind expects to find some relaxation and happiness there. If the mind is already feeling relaxed and happy, the senses lose their stranglehold on it and will not pull it to the external in search of relaxation. The resulting joy will impel us to further conquer our senses. One-pointedness allows the mind to overcome the senses. If we are able to conquer our senses, we can control our body and mind and achieve the desired results from our yogic practices very quickly and easily.

Only one who can control the senses is fit for Realization, and sense control arises through detachment and one-pointedness. These qualities can only arise when one's system is dominated by pure sattva energy. Pure sattva is possible only by practicing the principles of cleanliness. Hence, we see how the discipline of śauca paves the way for the final goal.

SANTOṢA: CONTENTMENT

The next niyama is *santoṣa,* or "contentment." Many people are confused about the difference between contentment and happiness. Contentment is a feeling of satisfaction, completeness, or being filled up in some way. Contentment arises from inside of us. It tends to have a lasting or enduring quality. Happiness is a feeling of pleasure or lightness that tends to be caused by some external source or for some external reason and is usually fleeting. Some examples may help to explain the difference.

Typically, a man will feel happy after he has acquired a new object or material that he has long desired. A man who is content, however, will feel the same happiness when he uses an object or material that has been in his possession for a long time. The first man will feel happy when he purchases a new automobile; the content man will feel happy when he maintains his old automobile so that it works reliably. While the first man will feel happy when he goes to a restaurant and eats delicious food, a content man will be deeply satisfied by simply preparing a flavorful dish in his own home.

CONTENTMENT COMES FROM WITHIN

The practice of santoṣa requires us to deeply assess, and realign, our core values. Contentment must be developed within. It is a capacity to feel happiness from what we already possess—both externally and internally. If our highest value is aligned with acquiring new materials, we will feel happiness only when we gain something new. When our highest value is aligned with living more simply and causing fewer disturbances, we will feel an even deeper happiness using fewer materials.

One of the attributes of a Realized person is contentment. Because he regularly experiences the highest bliss of Samādhi, he is completely satisfied with life; he is always content. Until we arrive at this point in our life, we will continue to crave materials, hoping that they will bring the contentment we seek. Instead, they bring only sporadic and temporary pleasure. As a result, we continue in a never-ending cycle, moving from desire to desire. As each desire is fulfilled, we experience a bit of joy and happiness, but never real contentment. When we are content, our continual search for gratification through external materials ends.

To reach Realization we need to develop santoṣa. The most important reason is that santoṣa helps keep the mind calm and quiet. How do we develop santoṣa? There are a few methods. First and foremost, contentment itself must be our goal and intention. We should recognize the value of cultivating contentment and the results that it brings to our lives. We must establish this as one of the important secondary goals in support of our primary target—Realization. Then we must cultivate dhṛti, or courageous determination, to achieve santoṣa in the presence of all obstacles.

CONTENTMENT AND THE INFLUENCE OF OTHERS

Yoga suggests that we should build friendships with people who are content. A few people have the constitution that easily supports this quality in their lives. They may be poor, have limited education, or even health problems, but still their nature is to be content. They always think positively and never dwell on their problems. They understand that their duty is to try and resolve their problems, but they take it easily if they cannot. They accept what life offers them, count their blessings, and are grateful for what they have. Such people are very happy; moreover, they are *content.* If we cultivate friendships with such people, their contentment will help engender this quality in our lives.

The difficulty with this approach is that it is rare to find such people. Nevertheless, we can find people who are somewhat content, and it is better to seek out their company than that of people who are always dissatisfied. When we meet those who are fully content, we should honor them and seek out their company.

EDUCATION

Another method for bringing about contentment is through education. What is the real purpose of education? True education enables us to understand the universe and how we might live a better life. By studying some suitable subject—science, mathematics, dance, or music, for example—students will develop an understanding of the world on many levels. As they learn their subject, a good teacher will bring a sense of balance to their minds and developing natures. Any one of sixty-four Indian sciences related to yoga, if properly understood, will develop balance in the minds of students and directly or indirectly lead to increased contentment.

A good teacher will closely observe each student. The student should be interested in progressing in her studies, while at the same time content with the knowledge she has gained. Her contentment should be balanced with *enthusiasm.* If the student develops an excess of contentment, she may become complacent and not progress to her fullest capacity. On the other hand, if she develops too much enthusiasm and proceeds too quickly, many problems may result. This can easily lead to disappointment or envy if the student expects to learn more than she is capable of learning. Therefore, maintaining a balance of enthusiasm and contentment is critical to reaching the goal of education, which is ultimately to learn how to live a better life.

Much of what passes for education today is no more than learning a technique to earn money, such as the operation of machinery or high-tech equipment. If education does not lead to the increased happiness of humankind, how is it worthwhile? Teaching about machines can be very beneficial if, at the same time, the teacher imparts knowledge that will bring balance to the student's mind and to the world. Of course, in today's world, a science instructor will rarely guide his students in living a balanced and contented life; but we should view this as a flaw in our system of education, rather than a flaw in our ideal.

A wise teacher should guide the student in cultivating contentment in all aspects of her life—health, money, possessions, relationships, knowledge, as well as her talents and limitations. This guidance is proper education. If education does not bring balance to the body and mind and lead the student to live a better life, it has failed.

Therefore, whenever possible, we should seek out teachers who are content themselves. The contentment of our teachers (or lack of it) will be transmitted to their students. This transference of important characteristics is one of the reasons we should be very careful about whom we ask to teach us.

LIVING WITHIN OUR MEANS

Living within our means is another way to develop contentment. After our formal education is complete, we get a job, earn some money, and proceed to live our lives. Each of us adopts a particular lifestyle. It may be simple, adequate, or luxurious. Too often, we set our sights on a luxurious lifestyle and then struggle to earn enough money to pay for it. What if we were willing to accept an interesting job that we could do fairly easily that generated less money? We then would have to make intelligent choices to create a simpler and more meaningful lifestyle. If we were to choose such an alternative, our struggle in life would be much less. We would find that happiness comes much more easily in other ways, and contentment would be our great reward.

With the money we earn, we can acquire the necessary possessions that allow us to live our lives. Ideally, we will be content with whatever amount comes to us by living a balanced way of life. If we work in a constructive way for eight hours, we earn a certain amount of money. When this happens easily, and without too much strain on our system or others', it is Nature's way of saying, "This is the allotted wealth for you." If we strain our system while attempting to earn more money, Nature is essentially warning us, "You are attempting to acquire more money than is in your best interest. You should stop and seek some other livelihood."

Sometimes an unexpected need may arise, and it becomes inevitable that we must work to meet that need. If our brother or sister gets sick and needs our support, it is our duty to provide support. If our child is ill and there is no health insurance, we need to provide the means to pay for the medical care. In these cases, we may need to work more than is natural to us. However, this should be the exception rather than the rule. We should not strain our system just to pay for an extravagant house or car. This is not to imply that our job should not challenge us. Challenge, within limits, is energizing, but the challenge should not be so great that it strains our system. Challenge is not the same thing as strain.

Out of the twenty-four hours of each day, eight are meant for working, eight for sleeping, and eight for yogic practice. Dedicating this much time each day to one's yoga practice may seem unrealistic, or even impossible, to many of us. However, depending on one's constitution and nature, duties like attending to one's spouse, children, and other family members may be incorporated into any one of these basic time allotments or be fulfilled on days of leisure. Also, many day-to-day activities may become part of one's yogic practice, providing one applies the yogic disciplines accordingly. This provides opportunities to practice the yamas and niyamas in all areas of our life.

WHAT IS WEALTH?

There is another way we might try to explain santoṣa. It is by asking the question, What is wealth? One answer is that which brings happiness. If this is indeed true, then instead of craving more money, or this or that material object, we would be far better off craving happiness itself. If we crave real happiness, we will try to understand and follow the principles by which happiness operates. If we are successful, we will automatically be wealthy. We will feel abundant happiness whether our possessions are many or few. If happiness is already present, there is no need for money or possessions. Our basic intention should be to find happiness, not wealth. If we succeed in gathering a lot of money and possessions, what are we going to do with them? Their real value lies solely in their contribution to our happiness. When we directly establish happiness in our system, we are already where we want to be. We are getting the full benefit of our wealth.

Regardless of our wealth, one who craves many things is poor, while one who is content is rich. Although one may be a king possessing an entire country, if he is filled with craving, he is poverty stricken. He always feels the scarcity of money and materials. In contrast, another man may live in a hut or a hermitage with very few possessions to sustain his life but crave nothing. He is totally content with what he has. This man is very rich, because he understands true wealth.

BUILDING OUR CAPACITY FOR SANTOṢA

If a mountaineer wants to ascend Mount Everest, he will prepare himself by conquering smaller mountains that are much less difficult to climb. Gradually, he will gain more experience and develop more skills. Then he will scale higher and higher mountains until he is ready to climb Mount Everest.

This is one way to approach our goal of Self-Realization. Self-Realization is the ultimate human experience and offers us the ultimate experience of joy and happiness. It is of the highest scale and intensity. The joy that one experiences in Samādhi is unimaginable. But do we have the capacity to bear this much happiness and joy? Most of us do not, until we develop it. How do we do this? Just as the mountain climber climbs progressively higher mountains, we must develop our capacity to feel more and more happiness. Contentment develops the capacity to experience this joy. Whenever we feel contentment in our lives, we build our inner resource to recognize and experience joy. Actually, any time we experience any form of happiness, it indirectly prepares our system to feel greater happiness. Joy begets joy.

As we progress along our yogic path, at each step we will feel some amount of happiness and joy. If we are able to bear that joy, we will be allowed to progress further. If not, our yogic path will be blocked. This blockage tells us that some hindrance exists in our system, either from our current birth or from a previous one. We have either committed an error or caused some imbalance that we have not yet corrected. We need to correct this in order to move forward. If there were no blockages in our system, we would immediately realize the Eternal Truth.

It is essential that we develop an increasing capacity to bear higher states of joy and happiness. As we develop the tendency to be content, there will be many changes in our system. These changes pave the way to enter into yogic experiences through different techniques. The yogic technique prāṇāyāma is one example. It is like a vehicle that has the capacity to transport us to our desired destination; its aim is to take us there. However, even though we may practice prāṇāyāma with intense dedication for years, some unknown obstacle can prevent us from entering the yogic state, and our system will remain unfit to enter. Conversely, if we first prepare our system to bear higher levels of joy and happiness, prāṇāyāma will move us to our destination easily. We will feel the maximum possible relaxation, calmness, and quietness of mind.

Contentment brings joy and happiness. These are all prerequisites for Realization. The greater our capacity for joy, the easier our progress will be on this internal path.

A COMMON MISUNDERSTANDING

There is a mistaken idea that contentment is detrimental to prosperity, that if we are satisfied with small things, we will lose our ambition and our desire to work hard; and the wealth of our family and country will be reduced. There is some truth in this idea. Some people appear to practice contentment without seriously involving themselves in yogic practice. They have sufficient time in the morning and evening, but they simply fritter it away and never sit for meditation. They distort the idea of contentment to justify an escape from work and their responsibility to their family and society. In fact, a closer look will reveal that these people are not really content at all. They often lack self-esteem and purpose in their lives. They are afraid to fully engage in life and have shirked all their duties. To justify their lives, they have twisted the underlying principles of santoṣa. This should be corrected through their own efforts or through the help of others.

True contentment does not lead to laziness. When we become firmly established in santoṣa, we work hard during the working hours, we practice diligently at the correct times, and we sleep soundly when it is time to take rest. Our goal is not to avoid work and human effort; it is to lead an ideal human life. It is the antithesis of laziness.

Moreover, true contentment does not lead to poverty. If we are content and happy, whatever we truly need comes to us with little effort. Over time, the more we see this principle in action, the more we learn to trust it. In fact, our prosperity will increase. We will enjoy life without worrying about acquiring the things that we need to live. This human body is made for happiness, and when we are happy, we bring balance to all of our surroundings. Animals, birds, and even vegetation will feel this balance and benefit from our happiness. We are richer because of their existence; they are richer because of ours. The whole of society may develop real wealth because of the contentment of a yogi.

OVERCONSUMPTION

A Realized yogi, who is established in the principles of contentment, will always be surrounded by wealth, and not only in terms of money. A contented yogi receives whatever materials he needs. He does not need to take ownership in order to benefit from their support, and so feels prosperous.

In contrast, those who acquire possessions through overwork and overambition often plunder nature. Their overconsumption may seem like wealth, but it brings imbalance to the universe, and this in turn brings nothing but unhappiness. Unfettered consumption has led to enormous problems in the natural environment, as well as throughout many societies. Dwindling natural resources, exploited labor, and a denigrated natural environment are all serious consequences of human beings not understanding the basic principles of santoṣa. Engaging in overconsumption thwarts our attempt to develop contentment and gain happiness from the wealth of Nature.

NATURAL VERSUS UNNATURAL DESIRES

We certainly need some material possessions, but need is different from unnecessary craving. Here we encounter the difference between natural and unnatural desires. Natural desires arise from an unconditioned mind. When we look at the world without filters, we soon realize that we have only a few needs. We will want to eat some nutritious and delicious food. We will want to see our friends and loved ones. We will want some suitable and appropriate clothing and adequate shelter or housing. We will also want a meaningful job to provide all these things. These things need not be oppressive and drab. We can enjoy them. Our clothes and our home may be functional and also beautiful. But we must be able to clearly discriminate when our desires become unnatural.

Unnatural desires are those that result from imitation of those around us. If we want something only because our neighbor has it, or because a clever ad campaign tells us we need it, or because we see it displayed in the mall, is it natural? Is it beneficial? These days, there are many advertisements everywhere. Their intent is to create unnatural desires. One such advertising principle is summed up in the saying "First hurt them, *then heal them.*" In other words, first make people feel that there is something wrong with them, and then convince them to buy a product to fix the problem. This is a cynical approach to marketing goods. We ought to ask ourselves whether noticing such advertisements and acting on their impetus will bring us the happiness we truly desire. We need to think for ourselves about what will really make us happy.

Our responsibility is to fulfill our natural desires, and to that end Nature will provide us with every opportunity we need. When human errors are prevalent across whole societies, and even nations, Nature will attempt to correct the imbalance. This is a result of all our collective karma. Small corrections occur constantly. For example, Nature constantly works to correct society's misuse of natural resources. When small corrections do not occur, an accumulation of energy may cause a huge imbalance that leads to a catastrophic event. Those who are trapped in those drastic corrections will receive the effects of this karma. Some may be injured, others may not get proper food, and others will be killed outright. The purpose of such drastic events is for this karma to unfold and thus bring balance to the planet.

Today, there are very few natural desires in comparison to the number of artificial ones. If we simply begin to eliminate the many artificial desires, we will begin to experience more and more happiness. Cultivating santoṣa works in harmony with eliminating these unnatural desires.

THE POWER OF MEMORY

There is another powerful method for cultivating contentment in our lives. After practicing yogic techniques for a period of time, we will feel a certain level of contentment, peace, and joy. If, the next time we wish to practice, we begin by simply sitting and recollecting these feelings, our memory alone will have the capacity to transport us directly to this state. We may then proceed with our yogic technique. It is even possible that we may be able to eliminate the yogic technique if we have mastered this skill of recalling our past experience. Any yogic technique is merely a vehicle to transport us to this place of peace and joy. In fact, remembering this thread of joy is the true technique. If we are able to reach yogic states through our memory of them, our need for practice is over; we can proceed using memory alone.

Another way we can develop this capacity is by remembering the happiness and joy in our life, whatever it may be, before we practice. This helps prepare our mind to move inward toward that great place of deep joy and contentment. We should sit and mull over these feelings, like a cow chewing its cud.

Sometimes contentment will come for no reason. By chance, at one point or another, we will be overcome by feelings of happiness and joy. Or, after a particularly fine sleep, we will wake up and feel an exquisite sense of well-being. These periods of internal contentment are important, and it is best to sit and memorize these feelings if possible. It may be helpful to keep a journal or small book to write detailed descriptions of these experiences. If we write in this book only when we are feeling very joyful, either naturally or because of the results of our yoga practice, it will support us in recollecting these wonderful feelings when we wish.

A clever aspirant uses the feeling of contentment as a thread to reach the Eternal Truth. Sometimes yogis use the analogy of a person who is lost in the woods. If there is a thread or string that leads out of the woods, we can find our way out easily, simply by following that thread. There are many threads we can follow to the Eternal Truth. When we cultivate and expand contentment in our lives, we create a thread that will gradually lead us to the supreme contentment of Realization.

TAPAS: AUSTERITY

The word *tapas* translates as "austerity" or "penance." The purpose of this practice is to help purify the mind and body so as to bring renewed balance to our system.

Each of us has deficiencies and impurities in our mind and body that can lead to external problems in our lives, like having too little money, no children, or an undesirable job. There are various external measures we might take to overcome these sorts of problems. Tapas, on the other hand, though they may be able to address some external problems, are generally reserved for the problems and imbalances that obstruct our yogic practice.

For example, sometimes a practitioner encounters problems in his meditation. His mind moves too much, or he falls asleep. Perhaps this discourages him from practicing regularly. Because of meager results, he is unlikely to feel much happiness from practicing at all and may soon lose interest. If this problem is not remedied in time, he may become unfit for yogic practice for the rest of his life. These kinds of problems are generally due to various imbalances, deficiencies, and impurities in the practitioner's system. In such cases, tapas is recommended. Practiced over time, certain tapas will eliminate these problems from our system, and desirable characteristics will replace them. The mind and body will become strong, stable, and focused. Unwanted traits like fickle-mindedness, laziness, and sleepiness will disappear.

THE DIGESTIVE FIRE

Tapas is also translated as "to burn." We cannot simply will away impurities from our system. But how do we burn such impurities? Burning requires fuel and a process: Impurities supply the fuel, and the digestive fire provides the process. The digestive fire possesses the characteristic of fire and burns whatever is within reach of its flames. Simply put, tapas is a method of provoking the digestive fire in order to consume the impurities in our systems.

Impurities need to dwell somewhere in our system. They will often attempt to hide in some basic component of our body and mind.

Āyurveda classifies seven basic components of the body called *dhātus.* These include plasma, blood, muscle, fat, bone, bone marrow, and sperm or ovum. But it may not always be easy to distinguish which components are deficient or imbalanced.

FASTING

In order to burn the impurities from her system, an aspirant practices various austerity measures, or tapas, which include chanting mantras, performing pūjas, and devotional singing. However, the primary form of tapas, highly encouraged by the sages, vigorously provokes the digestive fire by using food restrictions and dietary changes. When the practitioner reduces his food consumption, the digestive fire will seek to burn something else. When food is not provided, the digestive fire burns the impurities carried by the dhātus. This is how purification takes place during fasting.

Another dynamic comes into play when one experiences a strong hunger sensation. At that point, blood will flow from the external limbs to the internal digestive tract. Impurities will be carried with the blood to the digestive system, where they will be destroyed. In different types of fasting, for example, the practitioner might drink only one cup of milk per day and nothing else for an entire month. Alternatively, for sixteen days, he might drink only a few cups of water per day.

Yet another method begins on the day after the new moon. On that day the practitioner eats only one handful of food (about one bite), then increases this amount to two handfuls the following day, and so on up until the full moon. On the full moon, he eats fifteen handfuls of food and then reduces his food by one handful per day until the following new moon. On that day, he will not eat any food. This type of fasting is called *cāndrāyaṇa.*

SOURCES OF IMPURITIES

There are primarily two types of impurities found in our system. The first is related to karma and saṃskāra from our previous births. The second is related to our actions in this life. The impurities from previous births are very strong. Nature uses them to correct the practitioner through inevitable experiences of suffering. This may be corrected only to some extent through yogic practice.

Impurities from previous births need to have a physical root; they may come to the practitioner through his heredity. His Soul enters into a lineage where that particular impurity can come to his body. Externally, it looks as though the practitioner was just unlucky to be born to parents and grandparents from whom he inherited some physical deficiency or weakness, but really it has its roots in his previous births. He once made a mistake, and he will reap its consequences in this birth.

THE ROLE OF MĀYĀ IN TAPAS

Through the work of māyā, a practitioner's impurities will cover her mind so she will not recognize their existence. This covering may even cause the impurity to be seen as *purity,* and vice versa. This is why impurities are so difficult to overcome. As we explained about māyā, this delusion of the mind is by the grace of Nature. Nature wants to correct us. To achieve this end, Nature covers the mind in order to allow our saṃskāras to unfold. If we search by ourselves for our impurities, the mind will immediately move into some form of delusion, formulating an incorrect diagnosis. This type of delusion is seen in almost every human being. In Western psychology, this may appear as a form of *denial* or *self-delusion*.

For example, if a man is egotistic and quick to anger and we point out those qualities to him, he will likely protest in anger. He may even heatedly inform us that he is not egotistic, and that we have no right to confront him in this way. He does not see that his very response is a symptom of his egotism. This shows that he cannot identify his own impurities—primarily because egotism itself is an impurity that comes from karma and saṃskāra. To bring about eventual change, he needs to experience some suffering through the consequences of his past lives' errors. Thus, it is not easy to eliminate such an impurity.

Impurities may also be due to incorrect activities in this life. In each birth, we have a level of free will. With independence comes the potential to err that brings new impurities to the body, either in this birth or the next. If there is a possibility for them to be corrected in this birth, Nature will allow us to suffer the consequences immediately.

Otherwise, we will have to wait until a future birth. If the correction occurs in this birth, and we are able to recognize where we erred, the impurities can be eliminated much more easily.

REPENTANCE

We need to understand the damage that impurities in our system cause ourselves and others. Impurities exist because of our ignorance and other undesirable qualities. Our effort to eliminate them will be effective only when accompanied by sincere repentance. When tapas is approached in this way, our system will gradually burn the impurities. Furthermore, we will develop a greater tendency to avoid mistakes in the future.

FORMS OF TAPAS

Many books related to the ideal way of life prescribe an assortment of corrective measures devoted to the process of eliminating a variety of impurities from the body. These processes are all various forms of tapas. Many spiritual aspirants have used tapas to correct a physical disability, such as loss of hearing or sight.

Once there was a poet who was blind from birth. He wrote a famous poem that contained one hundred stanzas devoted to the sun god, who, in yoga philosophy, is closely connected to eyesight. During the writing of that poem, the poet prayed earnestly to the sun god to bless him with the sense of sight, which he had never known. His devotional praying, along with his steadfast commitment to his writing became this poet's tapas. Amazingly, the poet's eyes were corrected, and he could see. In India, there are many such instances documenting the beneficial results of using tapas. These kinds of transformations are possible, providing one uses the right practices and disciplines.

WORSHIP OR HONORING

Tapas may also involve serving and honoring some divine energy or deity. A story from the epic poem *Raghuvaṃśa* tells of a king named Dilīpa in the lineage of Rāma. This king and his wife, Sudakṣiṇā, were very religious. They followed all disciplines and never harmed anyone. Even though their lives were pure, they were unable to conceive a child. Feeling that having a child was part of their purpose on earth, they were very disappointed. One day they traveled to an āśrama where their teacher lived and asked him why they could not conceive. Their teacher, Vasiṣṭha, sat in meditation and was able to see the impurities in their bodies and understand their causes.

Vasiṣṭha saw that in a past birth, Dilīpa had once met Kāmadhenu, the wish-yielding cow, which is a divine energy that resides in each person's body. Yogis in Samādhi will often have a vision of this energy in the form of this deity. Whatever one asks of this deity will be granted.

However, though he met this divine cow, Dilīpa neglected to honor him. Because of Dilīpa's neglect, Kāmadhenu cursed him with the inability to have a child in the next birth. Vasiṣṭha suggested that Dilīpa and Sudakṣiṇā spend time honoring and worshiping Kāmadhenu's calf, Nandinī. They did so and eventually conceived a beautiful child.

TRANSFERENCE

Sometimes a noble and capable person can accept the transference of impurities from another person. For example, a practitioner devoted to making progress on his yogic path may be suffering greatly because of certain blocks and hindrances due to impurities. A Realized person may take on this person's suffering out of mercy or for other reasons. However, Nature supports such cases only if a precise technique is followed; otherwise, the transmission will not take place. Until a person possesses the physical and mental strength, as well as the education and knowledge of the proper techniques, he would be making a grave mistake to take on another's impurities. Better he remain focused on his own liberation first. Though there are aspirants and priests who accept such transference.

If the receiver of impurities is a Realized person, she will likely have the intention of carrying out specific missions while she is here on this earth. To do that, she may need various materials. The practitioner in need of transferring his impurities may have access to such materials and be willing to offer them to the Realized person. This is a type of rajasic offering: Each person offers something needed by the other. The practitioner makes his offering and moves on with his practice and his life. The sage will then need to perform austerities and penance to dissolve those newly acquired impurities. It is a very meaningful transaction, one that accords with, and is accepted by, both Nature and society. A loose analogy or rough equivalent in the West would be the psychological notion of transference between psychologist and patient. It also speaks to the materially rich Western student who may find some benefit in making material offerings to progress on their path.

CHANTING

One of the most famous poets of ancient India is named Kālidāsa. His own life story involved intense tapas practice when he was young. His story begins with a king who had a beautiful and intelligent daughter. The chief minister wanted the king's daughter to be the wife of his son. He approached the king about this plan, but the king refused, explaining that his daughter should marry a prince, not the son of a minister. While this may have seemed a harsh response, the king had many good reasons for his decision. Nevertheless, the minister felt insulted. He left angry and devised a scheme of revenge.

The minister went into the countryside and found a very handsome shepherd with the face of a prince. The shepherd was ignorant and uneducated, but the minister dressed him in the clothes of a prince and brought him back to the king's court. Through a number of tricks, he was able to hide the identity of the shepherd and presented him as a proper match for the princess. The king, the princess, and everyone in the king's court were fooled; and the king agreed to the marriage.

The shepherd was an honorable young man, and a victim himself of this great deception. He had not fully understood the fraud in which he was unwittingly involved. However, after the marriage, the couple realized the minister had deceived them. The princess realized that her husband was not a scholarly prince, but an uneducated shepherd.

At the time, once a marriage had taken place, it was considered unbreakable except in extremely rare circumstances. A difference of status and station between the husband and wife was not such a circumstance. Therefore, it was impossible to fix the problem by divorce. As the princess reflected on her situation, she realized that if she made public what had happened, it would be very disturbing for everyone. Her parents would be devastated; more important, the news might threaten the entire kingdom if proper succession was not assured.

As a result of these considerations, the princess decided to keep quiet about the matter until she could think of a better solution. Until then, she was committed to live as the wife of the shepherd. She understood that it would be impossible for her husband to learn all he needed to know. Even with the brightest mind, it would take far too many years for the shepherd to gain the knowledge of a prince. To solve her dilemma, she sought the counsel of a sage.

In his wisdom, the sage suggested to the couple, "Why doesn't this young man do a devotional practice whereby he may become a great poet and a learned man? He needn't read books or learn to write. He does not even have to listen to other scholars. Instead, he should simply devote himself to a practice of tapas."

The princess arranged for a suitable teacher to initiate her husband with a mantra associated with Sarasvatī, the goddess of learning. Her husband took that mantra into his heart and started chanting it regularly, with full devotion. His practice was a form of tapas, designed to address ignorance and lack of education. After some time, he gained the blessings of Sarasvatī and visualized her in his meditations. From then on, he gained enormous knowledge and grew to be a great scholar. In time, Kalidasa became one of India's most prolific and cherished poets, who went on to dictate many great poems, including *Raghuvaṃśa, Śakuntalā,* and other superb Saṃskṛta dramas.

IDENTIFYING IMPURITIES

The practice of tapas is very complex, and many questions will still arise: Since these impurities are so difficult to discern, how can we discover what they are? What austerities and penances should we perform to eliminate them? Often we cannot use our mind to diagnose ourselves; in general, the mind is unfit due to its own problems.

Fortunately, there are certain methods that can help us uncover the core of these disturbances. The best method is to ask a yogi to contemplate on our behalf. He may use his yogic sight, or he may have comprehensive knowledge about the body and mind, the nature of these impurities, their impact, their cause, and how we can eliminate them. In any case, he needs to be as skilled and experienced as a surgeon or a scientist. If it is not possible to find such a guide, we may even consult a Vedic astrologer. However, we should be careful. If this guide does not have real knowledge, we could be misled, waste our time, and perhaps damage our system. If we receive real guidance, however, certain practices can be offered to us.

SCIENCE OF TAPAS

In the past, whenever a student wanted to begin a yogic practice, his teacher would first study him to determine if he harbored any serious deficiencies and impurities. If the teacher concluded that there was a serious problem, he would advise the student to do tapas. The student would spend a few years performing these tapas to purify his entire system. This was a wonderful method of teaching. When the purification was complete, the teacher could impart his wisdom very easily, and the student would easily reach all of his desired goals.

Today, it is very difficult to carry out tapas in the prescribed manner. A novice should not perform such tapas without being fully educated. Yoga teachers and practitioners everywhere need to make it a priority to better understand the importance of tapas in their yoga practice. An aspirant must be prepared to use tapas, since everyone, knowingly or unknowingly, errs and acquires impurities in their system. The remedy for these errors is performing tapas. Some attempt to do these practices but often do not perform them in meaningful ways. Because of a fundamental lack of understanding, these aspirants will not gain the desired results. Attempting tapas without the prerequisite knowledge is simply creating more errors, the results of which they will have to reap in the future.

To do tapas meaningfully, many factors need to be in place. Until then, an aspirant should hold the concept of purification firmly in his mind. In addition, he should practice regular prayer for purification, along with right action and eating sattvic food act to purify the system. At some point in the future, an aspirant may have the opportunity, through the guidance of a true teacher, to do truly meaningful and beneficial tapas.

Patañjali himself prescribes tapas in the Yoga Sūtras, which later commentators define as *suitable, sacred,* and *measured food*—just as we have described mitāhāra. Properly selected food has the power to cleanse our system by helping burn impurities already in our body. It also prevents us from ingesting other food that might lead to additional impurities. This is a simple form of tapas that can be easily adapted by all aspirants.

In the past, much emphasis was placed on tapas. Today, the science of tapas has nearly disappeared, so these kinds of austerities are not practiced much, and yogic techniques suffer because of this. The exact mechanism of burning impurities is one of the mysteries that modern medical science has yet to explain. Few have a comprehensive understanding of these kinds of yogic techniques or the results that we should expect from them. Moreover, there is an equal level of ignorance about the hindrances seen in the body and mind. The mechanism of tapas may not be explained by allopathic medicine, but according to the testimony of many yogis, tapas is extremely effective in correcting deficiencies in the mind and body.

SVĀDHYĀYA: STUDY OF THE SELF

Who am I? What is the Soul? What is the universe, God, Eternal Truth? What is Realization? Liberation? What is bondage? What is this human body, and what are its components? How is it intended to best serve me? What has prompted creation? By what process does this universe evolve? Ultimately, how will this creation be merged into the Eternal Truth?

These are the questions we have been probing throughout this book. They are examples of what an aspirant seeks to understand in the niyama *svādhyāya*, or study of the Self. If we are able to grasp some basic answers to these questions intellectually, then we will better understand the full scope of the journey toward Self-Realization and Liberation.

PREPARING FOR OUR JOURNEY

Prior to embarking upon any great journey for the first time, we need to understand intellectually the challenges that lie ahead of us. For instance, if we want to cross a great ocean, we must consider many aspects of such a journey. What kind of boat will we use? Which route is best suited to take advantage of wind and ocean currents? What kinds of navigation equipment and provisions will we need? What kind of skilled sailors should be included in our party? In short, we should have enough information to be able to cross this ocean *mentally* before we set out on our physical journey. This is the practical knowledge we will need for our journey.

This is also true for our journey toward Self-Realization. Acquiring knowledge of the path ahead will prepare us to achieve the final goal. This knowledge is essential. If the path feels strange and unfamiliar, we may easily become fearful and hesitant to proceed at critical points along the way. If we are ignorant of the true challenges we face, our mind will likely reject what we need most to know.

Certainly, practical knowledge is important. For example, we need to understand something about food and its importance in cultivating an ideal way of life. We should know the steps for our prāṇāyāma practice. And we must understand some of the overall theory behind the science of yoga. A noble student will seek out the right source for this information—traditionally, a knowledgeable teacher—and apply herself seriously to the practice of svādhyāya.

A DIRECT APPROACH

There are many approaches to study of the Self. Aspirants should adopt an approach that suits their particular constitution and nature. For a few, like Ramana Maharshi, it will be possible to simply sit and contemplate on the Self, the "I" consciousness. For most, this technique is too challenging and will not yield results. If this kind of contemplation is to be successful, it requires a suitable constitution, extreme detachment, and intense interest in Realization.

As we explained earlier in the book, as the mind moves inward, it goes through a de-evolutionary process that returns it to its *causal states.* Manas, the externally focused mind, merges into its causal state, ahaṅkāra. This is where the consciousness of "I'" resides. Ahaṅkāra merges into mahat, or the bliss state, which merges into pradhāna, where total stillness of the mind is found. This is the state of Realization. This process is direct svādhyāya, or a direct approach to the Self.

THE VEDAS AND OṂ SOUND

Long ago, yogis received the Vedas, the oldest of Indian scriptures, as divine knowledge while in yogic trance, which is why chanting the Vedas is also considered a form of svādhyāya. The same is true for the Upaniṣads. If one studies these texts, and their underlying meanings, one will understand the universe and the Eternal Truth. However, due to the esoteric nature of how these texts were originally conceived, it is difficult for many readers to grasp their deeper meaning. Thus, it is better that one try to understand their meanings through oral teachings by a knowledgeable teacher. It is possible that the lack of proper understanding could hinder one's yogic journey. This is why such a path of study is not recommended for the ordinary person.

The Vedas are considered an evolution of the OṂ sound. OṂ is the sound form of the Eternal Truth, and it is considered a *Vedic mantra* (see "Mantra Yoga" in the appendix). By contemplating on this sound, an aspirant indirectly contemplates the Soul, or the Self. As with all Vedic mantras, the OṂ sound works most effectively as a vehicle when it is uttered with exact pronunciation. It has been thought that chanting this sound leads to an introverted nature and thereby does not fully support material prosperity. Hence, traditionally, the OṂ sound was chanted only by monks and other renunciates who had completely renounced the external world and whose sole intention was Liberation.

Nevertheless, each yoga aspirant has the potential to hear the OṂ sound at some point in her yogic journey. This occurs through an astral channel, or nāḍī. Hearing this sound pronounced incorrectly, however, may create blockages on one's yogic path. Some people will even attempt to shut their ears to avoid hearing someone pronounce the OṂ sound wrongly.

Thus, hearing and pronouncing OṂ should be considered a great responsibility. When one knows the science and value of something, his approach will be different from people who have little or no understanding. Each yogic technique has its own purpose and impact.

It is not advised to simply claim some technique at will. One should be guided and fully respect the disciplines surrounding that particular technique.

AN INDIRECT APPROACH TO SELF-STUDY

It is also possible to approach study of the Self indirectly. The study of yoga philosophy, for example, as laid out by Patañjali in the Yoga Sūtras, is a form of svādhyāya. Patañjali carefully and systematically explains who we are, what is the nature of the mind, what is Truth, and how we can achieve yogic conditions. It is a thorough and eloquent study of the Self. A teacher with a comprehensive understanding of these details will often encourage a student to start her yoga practice with this kind of study of the Self.

Some people are born into families that have a tradition of studying one or another of the sixty-four branches of Indian arts and sciences. These include Āyurveda, astrology, vāstu, sculpture, dance, music, poetry, cooking, and more. Any one of them can lead to Realization. Family members will often practice one of these, according to their lineage, as a form of svādhyāya. The constitutions of people born into those families are compatible with a particular art. Practicing it easily brings harmony and balance to their mind and body and indirectly supports their study of the Self. At some point, they will feel calm and quiet. They will gradually be able to understand their true nature and thus realize their true Self.

While the study of any one of these arts and sciences will lead an aspirant on the path of svādhyāya, some are more directly linked to this practice. For instance, to study the intricacies of food and cooking, we need to understand all the ways that food influences yoga practice. We need to know which foods propel us to move along the internal paths and which bring the mind to the external. We study how to eat, so that eating fully supports our primary target. If we study sculpture, we learn how sculpture is related to yoga. We study ways to avoid making sculpture that provokes the mind to the external and, instead, learn how sculpture can provoke the mind to move inward and experience bliss and happiness. If we study music, we study the effect of music on the mind. We come to understand which types of music bring about calm and quiet moods and facilitate meditation practice.

THE POWER OF STORY AND MYTH

Long ago in India, the public would gather near a temple in the evening, and a teacher would relate the tales of Rāma, Kṛṣṇa, and other great yogis. Everyone enjoyed these stories in a harmonious and relaxed atmosphere. The teacher imparted basic principles in terms that everyone could understand. Through telling these simple stories and mythological tales, a teacher could convey the essence of svādhyāya.

Some of the ancient sages had a vast amount of literary knowledge. In addition to being Realized, they possessed deep understanding about writing and the art of expression. Their voices were so powerful that they could enlighten almost anybody about important yogic concepts through their storytelling. Vālmīki and Vyāsa were such sages, who wrote the Rāmāyaṇa and the Mahābhārata, respectively. These two epics contain stories, both mythological and historical, that include many important principles that relate to all human beings. Listeners gained many important insights about humanity and gradually developed a greater capacity for inward contemplation. This is the power of story and myth. For many generations the Rāmāyaṇa and the Mahābhārata have provided essential teachings for all of humankind on the study of the Self.

Through the ages, it has become the duty of elderly family members to tell these stories to young children. There have been many examples of individuals whose spiritual evolution was a direct result of their mother, father, or grandparent sharing these wonderful tales at the child's early age. Even today, adults will sit together in the evenings listening to these stories when narrated by a skilled storyteller.

Effective storytelling is a very honorable task and the duty of one who possesses such a talent. A skilled storyteller understands how the mind of the listener works and how best to convey a story's hidden secrets. He will understand both what ails humankind and what remedies can heal. With a wonderful capacity of expression, he entertains, educates, tames, and even has the capacity to elevate the listener to states of higher consciousness. His storytelling is like a sugarcoated pill that can eliminate any problem and lead one to Self-Realization.

THE MAHĀBHĀRATA AND THE THREE GUṆAS

The Mahābhārata is an allegory for the human body. The universe, including our body, consists of the three basic energies, or guṇas: sattva, rajas, and tamas. The Mahābhārata is a story of the guṇas and how they interact with and attempt to dominate one another. It also clearly demonstrates their instability. It explains our duty as we sail in this ocean of energy (that is, the universe). It also guides us through the turbulence brought about by the constant flux of these energies. The three guṇas are interdependent, yet at the same time they display some competition with each other. At one point, sattva will dominate; after a few hours, tamas will dominate. Thus, we cannot always trust that sattva will be predominant. A clever person will do all in her power to continually give rise to sattva so that she can reach the goal of Realization as quickly as possible.

In the Mahābhārata, Kṛṣṇa leads the five virtuous Pāṇḍava brothers, students of Droṇācārya, against their enemies, the one hundred corrupt Kauravas. The Pāṇḍavas work diligently toward Liberation, believing that eternal happiness comes from contemplation of the Soul. The Kauravas, however, crave only the pleasures of the temporal world, believing that happiness can be gained through enjoyment of the material world. In the story, the Pāṇḍavas meditate on Kṛṣṇa as the representative of the Soul, or the Divine. They develop love and devotion for Kṛṣṇa and through that love realize the Self, or God. One of the lessons of the Mahābhārata is that those who have much devotion to Realization will win the battle, whereas those who are primarily interested in the external world will be caught by the cycle of birth and death.

The Pāṇḍavas represent virtue, and the Kauravas represent vice. Kṛṣṇa, as the Divine, supports the virtuous. This allegory represents the struggle between the virtuous and vicious energies in the body. According to the sacred Upaniṣads, our body contains 101 important astral tubes, or nāḍīs, that carry energy through the body. All but one of these nāḍīs moves primarily downward toward the external world.

The energy carried by those nāḍīs leads, directly or indirectly, to the next birth. If our energy travels primarily in those nāḍīs, we are forced to repeat the birth and death cycle. The allegory cautions us indirectly to disregard the nāḍīs that lead to the external and to focus instead on the one nāḍī that moves upward and to the internal. A person whose energy moves in that nāḍī will achieve Liberation.

The five Pāṇḍavas represent the five prāṇas, or energies that regulate our body. Prāṇa is life force. It is essentially one but splits into five in order to perform different actions for the various systems working in the body. These five are named *prāṇa, apāna, vyāna, udāna,* and *samāna*. Each of these five is located in a different region of the body. Prāṇa is situated in the heart center; apāna in the colon region; samāna in the navel region; udāna at the throat; and vyāna throughout the whole body. Among the five, prāṇa and apāna are the most important. Prāṇa is the energy that brings us to exhale; apāna brings us to inhale. These five prāṇas keep our system in full balance and allow us to experience both yoga and bhoga.

The Mahābhārata is largely about a battle between the external and the internal. The power of this story is to convey to the minds of many an indirect teaching of the Self. The Mahābhārata is also a vehicle for the teacher, or storyteller, to explain the underlying yogic philosophy in a manner that all can easily understand.

BHAGAVAD-GĪTĀ

The Bhagavad-Gītā is part of the Mahābhārata and is a vivid explanation of the creation of the universe, the voyage of a Soul through birth and death, the nature of duty, and much more. In very simple language, the Bhagavad-Gītā communicates the very essence of the Upaniṣads and the Brahmasūtra (philosophical aphorisms by the great sage Vyāsa). A powerful guide to the study of Self, the Bhagavad-Gītā offers an individual the necessary knowledge to always remain on the correct path, providing it is properly studied in depth.

Along with the Bhagavad-Gītā, a yoga practitioner with a firm practice of detachment may study the Upaniṣads and the Brahmasūtra. A lifetime of study would not exhaust the knowledge these texts offer. They contain all of the information we need to study the Self and thereby progress in our yoga practice. In this way, Patañjali's notion of svādhyāya parallels Yājñavalkya's siddhānta śravaṇa, which refers to listening to sacred readings and texts.

STAYING ON COURSE

While some study about the universe and the Self is essential for all seekers of Truth, sometimes, even with all this knowledge, one may be led off course. This is due to saṃskāras. Often when we are unable to follow the right path, we begin to sense, consciously or unconsciously, that we are doing something wrong and even counterproductive. This awareness will gradually help us. Eventually, we overcome such difficulties and set our path right. This is also why a teacher may offer knowledge to an ignoble person. Such a person may not overcome her saṃskāras in this lifetime, but if she realizes that she is heading for more suffering, she may be inspired to correct herself over time through meaningful repentance. If she does so, new saṃskāras will put her in a more favorable position in her next birth.

Those who practice svādhyāya reduce the disturbances in their body and mind, because they know what their target is and how they plan to reach it. Through this approach, practitioners can overcome many obstacles. According to Patañjali, the practice of svādhyāya will allow us to visualize a divine energy to support us on our path. This deity will help guide us and lead us to understand many things about our yogic path. We will keep our system in total balance and understand the direction in which we should move.

ĪŚVARA PRAṆIDHĀNA: SURRENDER TO THE ETERNAL TRUTH

Īśvara *praṇidhāna* means "surrender to the Eternal Truth." This is similar to what the sage Yājñavalkya calls Īśvara pūjana, the "worship of Īśvara," Śiva, or *God*. Once a student has studied some of the aspects of the universe, the Self, and the Eternal Truth, he should be convinced that the Eternal Truth is the supreme power in the universe. Understanding this, he develops an awareness of this Eternal Truth, and his attention then will never be far from it. As his awareness grows and deepens, it turns to devotion. This devotion results in Īśvara praṇidhāna, the surrender of all actions to the Eternal Truth.

DEVELOPING DEVOTION

Devotion to the Eternal Truth develops in a number of ways. One way is through study. When a practitioner begins on her path, she hears information from her teacher that gradually piques her interest and devotion. As her commitment to her yogic path matures, her interest and devotion become stronger. However, Īśvara praṇidhāna will reach its fullest extent only when the practitioner reaches Realization.

Another way devotion develops is through contemplation. Whenever we develop a new interest, or make plans for the future, we naturally become focused on our new activity. This is human nature. If we are moving to a new city, we think about which neighborhood will be best for us. We think about the climate and imagine how it will affect our life. If we have friends or relatives who live in that city, we make plans to see them. Similarly, if we are going to build a new house, we think about the features we want it to have. We may focus on the kitchen and imagine various ways of making it more convenient. We may plan where we want to place the windows and doors in order to take best advantage of the natural surroundings.

In this way, because an aspirant wants to realize the Eternal Truth, she focuses or contemplates on it. She thinks about how it will feel to be Realized. She imagines what she will see when she visualizes the Self. This contemplation is also a form of Īśvara praṇidhāna.

SURRENDER AND TRUST

When we feel that people are worthy of our trust, we naturally turn to them. We feel that their support provides us with something that we really need, so we depend on them. Eventually, we surrender ourselves to them. For instance, after a woman is married, the love for her husband will grow. When she feels fully supported by him, she will surrender to him. Likewise, when a man feels the love, affection, and support of his wife, he counts on her and surrenders to her. This is a natural tendency in all human beings.

In the same way, we gradually understand that our life force comes to us from the Eternal Truth, which exists everywhere and provides energy for all of our activities, both internal and external. When this Realization becomes well established, we naturally begin to surrender our actions to the Eternal Truth. We think, "I have done this work out of the energy that I received from the Eternal Truth, which exists in my heart. Because this energy came from the Eternal Truth, I want to surrender these actions to it." In the end, when we see the Eternal Truth everywhere, we will realize that all our actions are serving the Eternal Truth alone.

At the beginning of our spiritual path, we may practice Īśvara praṇidhāna somewhat mechanically. This may be our only option; it is not possible to force our own surrendering. A young child sees the actions of older people and pretends to be like them, doing what they do. When he grows older, his actions naturally become more authentic. Similarly, an aspirant hears his teacher speak of surrendering every action to the Eternal Truth. The student sees the attention and devotion that his teacher pays to the Divine and emulates this behavior. At some point, emulation becomes genuine behavior, and the student soon discovers what it means to truly surrender to the Eternal Truth.

A FLOW OF ENERGY

True surrendering of actions is possible only when we are doing our duty—when we are engaged in right actions that are in harmony with nature and the universe. The Eternal Truth is our source; it generously supplies energy for us when our actions are suitable and correct. The abundant flow of energy we feel as we are doing our duty is an indication that our efforts have been accepted. This flow of energy brings pleasure to us. Our enjoyment will increase as the flow of energy increases. This pleasure is a sign that we are properly creating a link to the Divine. It is this spark of divine energy that artists, athletes, teachers, scientists, and all people experience when their work is flowing to the ultimate extent. They are doing their duty. When we do our duty without struggle or expectation, it is easy to surrender the results of our efforts.

The universe has a particular intention for all energy, but if we use this energy for some other purpose, the Eternal Truth reduces the flow in our direction. If our activity is not suitable, it cannot be surrendered to the Divine. Unsuitable actions bring energy to the body in a twisted form, and we feel sad at the loss of the enjoyment we previously gained from doing our duty. Fortunately, this awareness can help us correct ourselves. When we direct more and more of our service toward the Divine, our sphere of service expands. We no longer imagine that we are serving merely our teacher, parents, friends, or relations; we perceive instead that we are serving the Divine itself. All right actions serve the Divine. This understanding will purify our system for Liberation.

DUTY AND RIGHT ACTION

Īśvara praṇidhāna has three benefits. First, it develops devotion toward the Eternal Truth. We will see the Eternal Truth in everyone and everything. Second, it develops right action. We will focus on attending to our appropriate duties. Third, it brings pleasure and enjoyment to our lives. But, in order to cultivate Īśvara praṇidhāna, we must be clear about what constitutes right actions and specifically what our duties are.

In the Mahābhārata, there is a story of a sage named Kauśika, a Brahmin whose elderly parents needed his help. But Kauśika believed that human life is best spent practicing austerities and doing penance in the pursuit of Liberation. So he left his parents and went into a forest to practice. Because of his great devotion, he soon attained certain yogic states and powers.

Then one day while he was out walking, a bird flew over Kauśika and released its droppings onto his head. Kauśika looked at the bird with rage, and the bird burst into flames and fell from the sky. Kauśika was astonished at what happened and began to feel proud of his new power.

At the time, sādhakas like Kauśika devoted all their time to their yogic disciplines. Instead of working, they begged for alms from house to house, living contentedly with the food they were given. One day, not long after the incident with the bird, Kauśika went to a house to beg for alms. But the housewife did not immediately answer his call from the gate. Her delay upset Kauśika. When she finally appeared at the gate, he showed his anger by glaring at her with piercing, penetrating eyes. Unaffected, the woman declared, "I am no bird." Kauśika was amazed and humbled by her awareness of the incident. He asked in astonishment, "How did you know about that?"

The woman replied, "I have understood this through my yogic sight."

It turned out that this woman was a yogini. She had an unconditioned mind because of the disciplined way she attended to her duties. As a result, she attained a small yogic siddhi, or power, which enabled her to read the minds of others. Curious about her powers, Kauśika asked, "How were you able to acquire this siddhi? What austerities and penances are you doing?"

The woman replied, "I am not doing any penance. I am only serving my husband as a housewife."

"Then how did you achieve this yogic sight?" Kauśika persisted.

The woman explained, "My husband is dedicated to the path of yoga and Realization. I am dedicated to him. This is my path. I achieved this power, as well as many other wonderful experiences, simply by doing my duty to my husband. When you came to my door, I was attending to him. This is my first duty. Attending to you was less important at that moment. Because of your egotism, you became upset. However, your angry eye could not burn me because I am shielded by the grace of the Divine."

The woman's dedication to her husband was not simply blind submission, but an expression of devotion to the Divine. This humbled Kauśika, and he asked, "Can you advise me about how to attend to my duty, so that I may become Liberated?"

The wise woman saw Kauśika as a half-baked pot. She did not advise him about his duties but aimed first to correct his egotism. She directed him, "If you really want to understand about duty, there is a shopkeeper in a village nearby. Go to see him, and you will understand more about duty."

Kauśika followed her directions and again was surprised. The woman had sent him to a mutton vendor. The sights and smells were repugnant to him. It was one of the last places he would have wanted to go, as he was a vegetarian and loathed to enter such a shop. Nevertheless, he approached the merchant.

Upon seeing the sādhaka, the merchant spoke, "Have you been sent here by the housewife?" Again, Kauśika was dumbfounded, this time to discover that the mutton vendor knew who had sent him. He asked, "Who are you? How did you know who sent me?"

The mutton vendor explained that he too possessed yogic sight and had gained his power simply because he performed his duty and followed prescribed disciplines. He added, "I am a butcher by birth. My father is also a butcher and required me to help him daily in this mutton shop. This is why I do this work. In a way, my father is like a deity to me. I also follow many disciplines in my life. Due to these things, I have attained many yogic experiences."

Then the mutton vendor admonished the Brahmin, "Your actions are misguided, and you have forgotten your duty to your parents. Though you are a dedicated practitioner and have acquired some yogic achievements, you will never achieve Realization if you do not perform your duty in life. Go home. Your father and mother crave your service. This is your first duty. Live in their house. It is also a sacred place to practice your yoga. Only then will your practice yield results."

Kauśika returned home to do as the mutton vendor ordered and served his father and mother. He also continued his yogic disciplines and in time became Realized himself.

This story offers a powerful lesson about Karma Yoga that leads us to Īśvara praṇidhāna. Performing duties is a fundamental part of yoga. When we do our duty, and surrender the results to God, we receive a flow of energy that supports our yogic path. When we are doing something other than our duty, our way forward will be blocked. In the case of Kauśika, sitting in a forest and meditating was not his first duty. His parents still needed him. The energy that he received by helping his parents was much greater than the energy he might have received by meditating in the forest.

Following the yogic path is just one among many duties. In fact, attending to our worldly duties can also be considered a yogic path, provided we approach these duties from the perspective of Īśvara praṇidhāna. For example, if a father and mother are suffering and need their daughter's help, their daughter can serve them as a yogic practice. While serving them, she should view them as representatives of the Divine, not simply as her father and mother. The Divine exists everywhere, including in the hearts of our parents. They are also the children of the Divine. We might think, "I worship the Divine through serving my parents. This is my duty. Through this service, I will reach my target."

When we understand our own constitution, we have solid clues as to what our duties are, including which actions are right for us and which are not. Right actions establish balance in our body and mind. That balance will allow us to recognize that when we have finished our duties, we will be ready to sit and meditate.

Traditionally in India, a person's work is determined by his heredity. Not everyone is suited to become a priest and worship the gods inside the temple. Someone must sweep the courtyard, tend the plants and flowers, and do other manual labor. The priest may achieve Liberation through his service in the temple. However, yoga affirms that the sweeper and manual laborer can also achieve Liberation through their work. Regardless of the work we do, our approach should be to think, "I am doing a service for all humankind, as well as seeking Liberation through my service. I can do this job well. I have a strong body and skills for these activities. My service will support the presence of the Divine." When we do our duty with this perspective, it gradually brings balance, as well as many other noble qualities to our system. Such qualities are prerequisites for Liberation.

SEEKING THE DIVINE IN OTHERS

If a close relation who is aging or sick asks us to dedicate a large amount of time to them, where will we find time for our yogic practice? There may not be any spare time left, so what must we do? We must serve them as best as we can, always keeping in mind that it is for the Divine inside of them that we do what we do. If we trust that we are supporting an instrument of the Divine, our service will reach God.

The same principle applies when practicing hospitality. When friends come to our home, we must view them as more than guests.

They are temples with God residing in their inner sanctuary. This is not mere imagery. They truly have the Eternal Truth in their hearts.

Thus, we recognize the link between those we love and the Divine. The next step is to feel this connection so strongly that we become fully immersed in it. Then we begin to see nothing but that connection. As we contemplate that link, day by day, we look for ways to make it deeper and stronger. This deep focus will bring many changes in our system.

This works in relation to other species, as well. A gardener can behold the Divine in each plant that he lovingly tends. As this link to the Divine increases, he will come to have faith in the reality of the soul in plants. If he contemplates the soul of plants, and his contemplation goes deeply enough, he will visualize the Eternal Truth.

THE LINK BETWEEN THE EXTERNAL AND INTERNAL

There are many ways to link to the Eternal Truth by attending to our duties, but it requires skill to catch the thread of the Eternal Truth that surrounds us at any given moment. How does this work?

As we surrender our actions, we receive energy from the Eternal Truth. This energy moves from the Eternal Truth to the external world through our mind. This energy paves the way between the Eternal Truth and this external world. Our mind must move on that same path when moving to the internal. As the energy comes from the Eternal Truth to the external, we can move to the internal easily on that same path. This may be experienced as a perceptible "thread" of bliss that, with practice and perseverance, our external consciousness can follow inward. The link between the external world and Eternal Truth thus becomes stronger.

We should be conscious of this dynamic, as it becomes more powerful when we are aware of it. This is true for all types of actions. If we do some physical work that is suitable to our constitution, we will feel meditative when we finish it. If we eat suitable food, our system will absorb it, regardless of whether we are practicing awareness. However, if we are aware that we are eating *sattvic* food, we can affirm, "This food is not tamasic. It will not make me sleepy. This food is not rajasic. It will not overly energize my body and make my mind fickle. It will support me with strong, clean energy that will allow me to sit quietly in a stable posture. This food will benefit my meditation." This food will then become a purifying force in our body, supporting our meditation.

The energy for all work and activities comes from the Eternal Truth. As that energy comes to us and returns to its source, it clears obstacles throughout our system. As a sign of this clearing, we naturally begin to want to be calm and quiet. Not only will it make us want to sit in meditation, it will also speed our achievement of Self-Realization.

There is a saying among those who practice yoga, "Work is worship." However, it is worship only if it paves the way between the external world and the Eternal Truth and allows for Liberation.

ĀSTIKYA: FAITH

Even if we have not seen or experienced the Eternal Truth, if we believe in its existence, it will be easier for us to reach the final target. This is *faith,* or *āstikya* in Saṃskṛta. However, yoga does not assert that we must blindly believe in order to reach our goal. It is possible to experience the Eternal Truth even without faith. Some yogic paths do not require faith at all; one simply needs to do the practice. At some point, the practice alone will yield its results, and we will understand what is authentic and true. Nevertheless, if we proceed with some faith, progress on our yogic path will be much more rapid.

Nobody lives without faith. Even outside the realm of yoga, faith is an integral part of human life. It is implicit in all of our activities. Even when we do something as simple as drink a glass of milk, we have faith that the milk is not poisonous. When we board an airplane, we do not test to make sure that the laws of aerodynamics still hold true. We will not double-check to make sure the plane has enough fuel for our trip. It is impossible for us to know everything about all the aspects of the world we depend upon each day. One cannot live without faith; we operate with faith every day of our lives.

Animals, too, display a kind of faith in how they live their lives. They do not worry or doubt that they will find enough food to eat each day. Nor are they overly concerned about the future. Even though many will build homes, and even collect and store food, they live with confidence and faith that their lives will go smoothly.

DOUBT AND HESITATION

Imagine that we want to travel to see a beautiful lake in the mountains. A friend of ours is well acquainted with this place and has given us directions. If we accept his advice, we will go with a level of confidence and proceed directly to our destination. However, if we worry that we may have the wrong information, our journey will be filled with doubt and hesitation, and our uncertainty will cause delay. If we accept what sound information exists, we can proceed as though we are fully certain of our goal—even if we do not yet fully know that information to be the truth.

If we accept the principles of reincarnation, for another example, we begin to understand the underlying reasons for many incidents in life. If we accept the idea of karmic impressions from previous births, not only will we be very careful in our actions, we will find many solutions to our problems. In this way, we accept some things to be true, even though we have not personally confirmed them.

Faith is an honorable quality. It should be well established in each of us. It is essential at many levels of our existence. At the same time, faith should never be "blind" or based on ignorance. Through direct perception, inference, and testimonials, one must try to understand the Truth to the maximum extent. One must inquire and try to find answers to one's own doubts. Blind faith may cause tremendous damage. My Eternal Teacher, Śrī Raṅga, used to say, "Faith built upon wrong concepts will not lead one to his goal. Rather, faith should be based in something meaningful. If we have faith that a road leads to the north, and in actuality it leads to the south, we will never reach our destination."

We must therefore place our faith in the appropriate tools of understanding—such as karma and reincarnation—to see real results. In order to select the right tools, we can either use those that have been time-tested by others, or make our best effort to assess their appropriateness. Through the use of these tools, we should inquire into the Truth with our best effort, after which we should have faith in our teachers and guides.

If we accept the Eternal Truth, changes will occur within our system that enable us to more readily visualize it. Those who do not have faith will experience a slower rate of change in their mind and body. Those who do not believe have no target; thus, doubt becomes a hindrance in their system.

STUDY OF THE SELF AS A PATH TO FAITH

Āstikya is closely related to aspects of svādhyāya, as well as the niyama we will discuss at the end of this chapter, siddhānta śravaṇa, or listening to the Truth. These three disciplines work in harmony with one another. When we hear more and more information about the Eternal Truth from a Realized person, or through yogic teachings and texts like the Upaniṣads, it becomes easier to have faith. This also brings changes to one's system. One will always gain more from one's learning, however, if one is able to believe in the Eternal Truth while learning about it.

Faith supports us and helps us to avoid dead ends. It will prepare us to visualize the Eternal Truth. Because of this, it is advantageous to believe. But we need not forever rely on faith alone. At some point in our practice, we will experience the Eternal Truth. Then we need not merely believe, for we will have seen.

DĀNA: OFFERING

The biggest obstacle on the yogic path is attachment. If we try to send the mind inward, it may refuse to go because of our attachment tendencies. The mind fears losing objects to which it is attached, so it wants to look at and engage with them constantly. It wants to experience and enjoy them. The root problem of any practitioner is that his mind drags him toward the material objects to which he is attached. This is the basic problem with human beings. If we had no attachments, we could easily achieve Realization.

How can we lose our tendencies of attachment to this material world? This is a fundamental question facing all aspirants. There are two basic approaches to answering this question. The first is through education.

As we gain greater understanding, our attachment diminishes. A small child is attached to toys, but as she grows and learns, she naturally loses interest in them. In the same way, when we become educated about the true value of materials, the true value of human life, and the true value of the Eternal Truth, our attachment tendencies lessen.

Another approach is to cultivate the practice of *dāna,* or "offering." Giving, sharing, and offering are signs that we are experiencing a level of detachment. Those who have fewer attachments have a tendency to make these gestures of generosity. When a person is very attached to his worldly materials, it is difficult for him to be truly generous. Either he is unable to make an offering, or he expects something in return. If we have fewer attachments, we make offerings naturally. Simultaneously, when we cultivate generosity, it reinforces detachment.

NATURAL GENEROSITY

Generosity is a noble quality. It opens the mind and heart to appreciate this universe and all that it encompasses. As a token of appreciation, one will think of the welfare of others. One will sincerely desire to help in whatever way one can, be that through money, materials, physical effort, words, and so on. At the same time, because of this deep appreciation, there is no expectation of receiving anything in return.

Generosity is a natural quality for all human beings, one that many people are endowed with from birth. Many families see this quality passed along from generation to generation. However, due to basic ignorance and attachment tendencies, the quality of generosity is often buried. Only through education and self-inquiry can it be brought back and nurtured once again.

Those who are truly generous are endowed with certain graces of Nature. They are seldom attacked and rarely troubled by jealousy or pride. They are well balanced and often have plenty of money and worldly materials for their enjoyment. There is a saying in Saṃskṛta that states, "For a generous man, the earth is his house and all living beings his family."

ATTACHMENT

Nature will offer us many boons and blessings if we are fit to receive them. But some will be deprived of these offerings primarily because of over-attachment, which blocks certain parts of their system so they are unable to receive Nature's grace.

This is not a metaphysical or mystical dynamic. It is simply common sense. If we are overattached in some area of our life, we will not be paying proper attention to other areas and will miss opportunities in those areas. Some opportunity may be calling to us, but we cannot hear it. For example, a man may be overly attached to his work or money. He constantly focuses on working more, how to gain more money, and how to keep the money he has. At the same time, he may desire to get married and live with his wife to create a happy home. Even though he is physically and emotionally ready for marriage, because of his focus on work, he will neglect that area of life. Even once he gets married and has a child, he may not give his family proper attention. Tragically, his overattachment to one dimension of life may prevent him from experiencing much greater happiness and fulfillment.

If we understand the purpose of life, as well as the purpose of materials, many opportunities will open to us. These opportunities are always available, but they require the knowledge of certain principles to see them.

For instance, many of the imbalances in our bodies occur because we lack some essential gifts of Nature. Our body has certain needs, and Nature constantly offers to fulfill them, but our attachment in some area can block our ability to receive them. A person may be in need of fresh air and exercise for her body, but because she is attached to watching television, she will not take advantage of what Nature freely offers. If we know the purpose of our body, and if we attend to its requirements instead of grasping after unnecessary objects, many of our problems will be solved. We will develop fitness for Liberation. But how can we truly meet our body's requirements through the bounty of Nature?

THE GRACE OF NATURE

Nature wants to constantly offer its bounty of goods and materials freely. These come in a multitude of ways and forms. They range from natural objects of beauty, to foods and items for our sustenance, to synthetic materials everywhere and even money. Nature uses us as a conduit to distribute materials everywhere. If a person does not become attached to those materials, Nature will flow materials through this person. As a result, this person will receive more and more of Nature's bounty.

The more this bounty is shared, the more it grows. We can easily see this in the way plants and flowers multiply. They freely offer their fruits and seeds; in doing so, their seeds are distributed and the plants grow more abundantly. The same occurs with our own body's fitness and physical strength. If we do not use our body wisely and offer its strength purposefully, we will lose its fitness. Likewise, when we share our knowledge with others, we learn from others. This meaningful exchange is a natural phenomenon.

THREE TYPES OF OFFERINGS

When we make an offering, or a gift, Nature offers something back to us. We have one set of needs; someone else has a different set of needs. One of our assets may fulfill one of that person's needs. If we offer a gift where it is needed, then what we need may be offered to us in return. With less attachment, we begin to see the offerings of Nature with an unconditioned mind. We will be open to receive these offerings, enjoy them fully, and then easily let them go.

The three types of offerings are *tamasic, rajasic,* and *sattvic*.

Tamasic Offering. A *tamasic offering* is one that we give in ignorance. For example, we may not know the real value of the material we are offering or whether the person is even fit to receive our gift. Or we may offer something and not know whether it will be used for a good purpose. At times, someone asks for something—such as money or other materials—and we give it without properly understanding whether it is the right time and place for us to be sharing such a thing.

For example, if a man has a tendency to overeat, and we offer platefuls of delicious food to him, he may overeat and end up with even more problems. Or we might feel compelled to give money to a beggar on the street who then uses our offering to buy alcohol, thus causing further harm to himself and perhaps others. Our offering may cause more harm than benefit. It can be difficult to assess the effects that our gifts and offerings will have on recipients. Therefore, we should be careful. An offer that arises from ignorance may well be a misuse of wealth.

Rajasic Offering. A rajasic offering occurs with the intention of an exchange. If this is done in the open, it is a business. It goes like this: "We want to purchase some goods from a store. We have money. The store has what we want." This is very direct. This type of exchange is beneficial. For instance, even a simple life requires many types of physical materials, such as food and clothing, for basic sustenance. If we cannot grow food or easily walk into the forest to find it, we need to depend on someone else to provide it. In an equitable exchange, we get what we need, and we offer something in return.

Sometimes an offering may appear to be a charitable contribution, but in reality it is a type of business transaction. One person is offering something to another. It looks like he is offering it freely, but in truth he is expecting something in return. This has a detrimental effect, because if the receiver is not able to understand the intention of the giver, he runs the risk of offending the giver or finding himself in debt. This is not a beneficial offering. Either the giver should speak frankly, explaining that he is giving with the expectation of something in return, or he should not expect anything in return.

These days, many rajasic offerings are made as a result of distorted thinking. Those who are offering are not properly educated in the skill of straightforwardness. For instance, someone may invite a guest to his home for a meal, but with the covert intention of getting financial support for a business venture or for his favorite cause. Similarly, he may intend to develop friendship with someone for an ulterior motive. Sometimes a friend will invite us to his home for food with an expectation that we will reciprocate at some point. This is not that harmful, but it nonetheless is an offering that comes "with strings attached." In such a case, we should simply offer a meal in return. If it is pure business, it should be called business; if it is a charitable offering, it should be called as such. We should not confuse the two.

Sattvic Offering. The third variety of offering is *sattvic*. It has several characteristics. First, the offering is given to someone who is going to use the benefits, such as money or materials, in a positive way. The proper material is given to the right person at the right time and place. Second, it is given without any conditions. The giver has no expectation of getting anything in return. The receiver may help the giver, or she may not. Ideally, the gift will spread out to any worthy place in the universe. The giver also has no expectations about how the material will be used by the receiver. Finally, the offering should not be a burden for either the giver or receiver. It should be something that can be easily offered and accepted.

A sattvic offering brings wonderful results in many ways. First, it develops detachment. Second, it helps a worthy person and therefore establishes balance in the universe. Third, the one who offers will also benefit from the support of the universe, though there is no expectation of this.

We will begin to recognize that we have made a sattvic offering when we feel a flow of joy. As the energy of Nature flows through us, not only will it convey materials to the right people around us, it also brings joy. That flood of happiness is our assurance that our offering is going to the right place and will not be wasted.

NATURE'S GIFTS

Nature supports those in need in two ways. One is by using a knowledgeable person who is totally conscious about the principles of offering. Or Nature may use a person who is unaware of those principles, but who acts as an intermediary to distribute wealth to a deserving person. The intermediary unknowingly becomes the medium of Nature. An unknowing person may be provoked to acquire some material and by chance offer it where it is needed. In this way, Nature compels the unaware agent, who will act unconsciously.

Nature constantly offers blessings. For instance, if we sow a seed, it grows into a tree and provides fruit, as well as hundreds more seeds. Through that first seed, we are offered fruit. Through the rain, we are offered water. Through the wind, we are offered fresh air. Nature is constantly offering us her bounty. Even the immense destructive forces of Nature—earthquakes, floods, volcanoes, tsunamis—ultimately offer renewal and rebirth brought through destruction. We cannot live without Nature.

The practice of offering is natural for a healthy human being. Procreation is a type of offering, one of many made by our parents. At the beginning of life, a mother offers her womb and a father offers his sperm. When two people properly conceive a child, many favorable conditions must be in place. The parents should be practicing disciplines to help prepare their bodies so that they are fit to conceive. A child should be conceived at the right place and time. When parents conceive in this fashion, with the help of Nature, they will have a noble child who may be suitable for Realization. This will fill them with joy and happiness. They will intuitively feel that they are Nature's means for bringing this Soul to the world. This is a sattvic offering. As with any other sattvic offering, the parents' happiness is due to the flow of Nature's energy through them.

Through the grace of Nature, we have received our body, mind, and senses from our parents. What we see, hear, and touch are all offerings to us from Nature. The knowledge that we gain from our parents, as well as the information and knowledge that wise people share with us, is also an offering. Nature constantly offers, and we are constantly receiving. Being part of Nature, this practice of offering should come naturally to us.

If we are grounded in the principles of dāna, Nature will use us as a medium to offer the Divine's grace throughout the universe. Nature is always searching for fit, noble people to serve as conduits for this grace to flow. Such people value all gifts from Nature and recognize their benefits when used in a proper way. If a certain material brings blessings to the universe, we must not hoard it unnecessarily. On the contrary, when we make an offering to the right person at the right time, we may begin to notice an increasing flow of materials from Nature passing through us to appropriate people and places in our lives.

HRĪHI: MORAL CONSCIENCE

As we have explained throughout this book, the human system is intended for Realization. This is our original nature, but it is possible only when there is a deep understanding about our duty to cultivate, possess, and protect noble qualities like nonviolence, truthfulness, nonstealing, contentment, and so on. These noble qualities will be found more or less according to one's constitution. They are gifts of Nature and lead us toward Realization. If we protect our original nature, we will not be disturbed by negative outside influences. We are also naturally endowed with a kind of shield to protect and guide us on our yoga path. This shield underlies the niyama *hrīhi.* As our *moral conscience,* hrīhi keeps us aligned with our own true nature.

Hrīhi may also be understood as a type of remorse or regret. When we act inappropriately, we feel remorse or regret for our misdeed. If we know that others are aware of our wrongdoing, these feelings are magnified. A certain retraction of the mind and body moves us to avoid wrongdoings. This moral conscience is evident in all healthy human beings.

Hrīhi also refers to a certain shyness and restraint. Wrongdoing is one of the obstacles to yoga. For instance, a yoga student who has achieved a measure of success on his yogic path has done so through practice and the grace of his teacher. At some point, he may become egotistical. Let us say the teacher makes a request and the student refuses to comply. Or the student may neglect or even insult his teacher. If such a thing happens, the student may lose his yogic achievements, because the growth in his system is mainly due to his teacher. When there is a misunderstanding between the student and the teacher, the yogic path for the student is blocked, and it will not be possible for him to reach his goal. If a student has a reserved nature and is capable of feeling healthy shame, however, he would never think of insulting or causing a problem for his teacher. If the student does not have such a nature, mistakes are inevitable. Therefore, all students should cultivate mature restraint, which will shelter them from wrongdoings.

That is not to say that a noble student should be timid. During the student's education, he will learn to understand the difference between right action and wrong action. A noble student develops an aversion to wrong action, and at the same time develops enthusiasm for right action, known in Saṃskṛta as *utsāha*. Hrīhi is the mature discrimination that knows the difference between these two.

MATI: INTELLECTUAL CONFIDENCE

Mati is a discipline to develop confidence in our intellectual abilities when applied to the science of yoga and Liberation. An aspirant who becomes firmly established in mati understands the correctness of the practices, rules, and regulations set down by the sages. An essential aspect of mati is the sense of confidence, or faith, that an aspirant develops due to the right functioning of his intellect. While āstikya is faith in the Eternal Truth and the teacher, mati can be understood as faith in one's own intellectual assessment of the teachings and techniques taught.

The most important principle for right action is an unconditioned mind. An aspirant may have questions at first about some of the practices recommended by his teacher. He may not be fully convinced about the importance of various principles found in the yamas and niyamas. In either case, his teacher may give him additional guidance and information. If the aspirant has an unconditioned mind, he will easily assess this information and become convinced. Correct intellectual assessment is an example of mati.

On our spiritual journey of Realization and Liberation, one of our primary tools is our intellect. If our intellect operates in a faulty manner, there is no limit to the problems it can cause us. If our intellect works well, fewer obstacles and hindrances will beset us. As an example, during the first six months of practice, sattvic vegetarian foods are most favorable for serious practitioners. An aspirant with mati will grasp the value of this and adopt these foods into his diet.

AN ESSENTIAL TOOL

When a practitioner attempts to understand Nature and the principles that govern it, a good intellect is essential. A good intellect will help him resist doubts about the path. He need not research every detail about each limb and attempt to reach a conclusion about each one. Having come to a general conclusion about the path, he can set many details aside and contemplate fully on Liberation. However, if he is unable to develop intellectual faith, he will need to assess each recommendation along the way. He will waste an enormous amount of valuable time, and his doubt will become his burden.

Some students become overly focused on philosophical inquiry, but once a certain level of understanding is achieved, a mature aspirant will begin to naturally surrender doubts and craving more information. He develops faith and confidence on his path based on his growing maturity. Through faith and confidence in the principles, the aspirant will achieve faster and better results on his yogic path.

FAITH, TRUST, AND CONFIDENCE

Once a student takes a teacher, and once the teacher accepts the student, confidence in the teacher is the same as confidence in this yogic path. Before taking the teacher, the student will study the teacher and come to an intellectual conclusion about him. Then the student is encouraged to develop mati about his teacher. For example, a yoga teacher may tell a student to go live at a particular spot and practice because that spot suits the student. If the student has faith and confidence in his teacher, he will immediately follow his teacher's instructions. If he has serious doubts, he will investigate his teacher's recommendations at length. He will wonder if he should trust his teacher. He may perform many experiments. During the time he spends questioning his teacher, he will not be making progress on his path.

When our intellect works correctly, it naturally develops trust in the authentic. This intellect-based trust is not just for the yogic path, it is seen in many fields of endeavor. When scientists investigate a phenomenon, we trust their findings. Or we feel it necessary to analyze their report and determine whether they are to be trusted. Perhaps we might even research other sources to verify their results. Then, like the student who first studies his teacher, we develop more trust and confidence in their work and their scientific conclusions. We function in the world with a new level of confidence in relation to their scientific work.

DEVELOPING RIGHT INTELLECT

An unconditioned mind means an undisturbed mind, free from erroneous thoughts and conclusions. When the mind is not polluted with wrong thinking, it works well. The keys for having a balanced mind are right work, good rest, correct food, and a predominance of sattvic energy throughout our system. Furthermore, eliminating unnecessary activities aids us in developing right intellect. There is a mistaken idea that one whose mind is constantly moving and thinking is one who has a good intellect. Such a person will have many thoughts, but she will be less likely to assess whether those thoughts are correct. In contrast, one who lives in as quiet a manner as possible will have fewer thoughts, but those thoughts will more often be correct. Rest for the mind keeps it in right order and allows us to more easily trust our decisions.

FOOD AND INTELLECT

If we use food to provoke and nurture sattvic energy in our system, our mind will enjoy improved functioning. If we experience too much tamasic energy because of something that we ate, our mind will be dull, sleepy, or deluded. It will not be able to pierce the core of the matter, so we will not feel confident in our assessments. If we eat highly rajasic foods, our mind cannot slow down enough to see which of our many thoughts are correct. On the other hand, a person with a sattvic mind observes something in nature, comes to a correct conclusion about it, and feels confidence in the assessment he makes. In addition to food, many of the disciplines associated with purification provoke sattva. Yogis recommend that we practice such disciplines to bring the intellect to a right condition. When we cultivate faith and confidence through right intellect, our path is smoother and our way is easier. This is the essence of mati.

JAPA: CHANTING

All Saṃskṛta syllables are associated with specific centers of the body. Words are formed from these syllables. If they are chanted perfectly, the mind develops the capacity for contemplation on that particular center in the body. If the mind contemplates more and more deeply, then it is possible to fully open a yogic channel from that center and become Realized. This is *japa*, or "chanting." Japa is a form of Mantra Yoga.

MANTRA YOGA

Sounds have an enormous impact on our system. Heard regularly, certain sounds develop noble qualities; others develop ignoble qualities. During worship, Hindus often use the sound of certain bells designed to imitate the sound of OṂ to invite positive and noble energies and eliminate negative ones. This is true of other sounds, as well. Music sung by someone with a beautiful and melodious voice may raise noble thoughts, of such things as mercy, generosity, peace, happiness, calmness, and so on. The sound of someone's voice carries this power and much more.

Making sounds and having the ability to talk are truly two of the most fantastic miracles in the universe. Sages tell us that this ability to talk, to make sounds that have meaning, is not a random accident of nature. Rather, it has been divinely and intentionally granted for our use and benefit. It is an integral part of this most miraculous creation: the human being.

Yoga philosophy explains that each material in the universe has evolved from a particular energy. These energies arise from the spirit world, sometimes called the *astral world*, and are each associated with a particular sound. Each *energy* has a *sound* and a corresponding physical manifestation, or *material*. In other words, each physical object in the world, its energy, and a particular sound are all inextricably linked.

A sound contains a link to its source. Like a vehicle, a sound can transport a practitioner to its root. A sound that is associated with the Eternal Truth can guide us to that Truth. A sound that is associated with a deity, or divine energy, can invoke a visualization of that energy or deity. Sounds that have this capacity to lead us to their origin are considered by yogis to be good for chanting. This is what is meant by *mantra*.

Yoga philosophy explains that the source of this entire universe, the Eternal Truth, has the sound form Oṃ. When the Eternal Truth evolved into the universe, it split into two parts, prakṛti and puruṣa. The creation of prakṛti, or all that is manifest in this universe, evolved in twenty-four stages. The male energy of prakṛti creates the physical universe; the female energy of prakṛti is the source of sound associated with the physical universe. As part of this evolution, Oṃ evolved into fifty sounds or syllables—forming the basis of the Saṃskṛta alphabet. These syllables then combined with one another to form words. Thus, through these steps of evolution, both materials and their corresponding sounds (words) were created and linked. Hence, there is a natural word for every material. They are like the two sides of a coin, inseparable.

When we look at anything in the universe, we normally see the material side of it. But by concentrating deeply on a material, it is possible to ascertain the energy of that material, as well as the word associated with it. Though these words are not heard by our external ears, they are heard through internal yogic listening.

Through this kind of listening, yogis are able to access the source of various divine energies while in Samādhi. Many people have misconceptions about deities and the divine world, often due to misunderstood religious teachings and imagery. Deities are manifestations of this divine energy and can be found everywhere in the universe, including our human body. Many people have misconceptions about deities and the divine world. These divine energies are invoked when a particular sound, or combination of sounds, are chanted. For example, deliberately uniting the syllables *ra* and *ma* creates a particular sound form that invokes a particular center of energy within our body. These sound forms are mantras. Great yogis in the past taught these sacred sounds to their disciples and established the tradition of Mantra Yoga.

TWO BRANCHES OF JAPA

There are two branches of japa—Vedic and non-Vedic, or *laukika*. In the ancient literature of the Vedas certain words and sentences, such as OṂ and GĀYATRĪ, are sacred. Chanting these words and sentences is *Vedic Japa*. Sometimes these words and sentences will be taught to a student for his contemplation, but, as we pointed out earlier, it is advised that they be chanted with exact pitch and pronunciation.

GĀYATRĪ

The GĀYATRĪ mantra evolved out of the OṂ sound. GĀYATRĪ is known as the king of mantras and the mother of the Vedas. The Vedas are considered to have evolved out of GĀYATRĪ. Like the OṂ sound, GĀYATRĪ requires certain disciplines to release its effects. It should be chanted after a bath, when one is wearing fresh, laundered clothing. This clothing should not be cut or stitched, as this is considered disturbing to the flow of energy throughout the body. One should sit on a mat, or wooden pallet, facing the East or North. Then the mantra must be chanted with full honor, followed by meaningful prayers.

Today, GĀYATRĪ is sung and pronounced in many undisciplined manners. This may leave wrong impressions in both those who are chanting and those who hear the chanting. This is because the sound does not properly invoke the corresponding center of energy within our body. This misguided experience may leave a lasting impression that blocks access to this energy in the future. This is largely because the wrong pronunciation and the music itself become a distraction to one's meditation practice. As a result, this unique yogic path may become spoiled for sincere aspirants.

LAUKIKA JAPA

When a student is not capable of pronouncing these syllables, words, and sentences exactly, or is unfit for Vedic chanting, he is taught laukika, or non-Vedic, mantras that work through devotion alone. Here it is the student's devotion that works to deepen contemplation, thus developing an awareness of the Divine. Examples of non-Vedic mantras are "NAMO NĀRĀYAṆĀYA" and "NAMAḤA ŚIVĀYA." The student may chant these for long periods. The pronunciation and sound of the chant are important, but even more important is the devotion. This devotion focuses the mind on some deity, such as Śiva, Viṣṇu, or Gaṇapati. The aspirant's approach should be, "I salute Śiva. *I want to visualize him.*" Through depth of devotion and contemplation, at some point the aspirant will visualize that deity.

THREE METHODS TO PRACTICE JAPA

There are also three different methods to practice japa, regardless of which branch one is using. The first method is to chant very loudly. This is what is seen in some āśramas, where aspirants chant loudly and with great devotion. The second method is to chant softly. And the third method is to chant the mantra silently, or *mentally.*

Loud chanting is meant to influence the external world, but in the context of Realization, it is the least powerful. Some texts estimate that chanting softly is one thousand times more powerful than the loud method. The mental form of chanting is said to be one thousand times more powerful than the soft method. The reason is that while we are producing actual sound, our body and mind are more active. Yogic achievements are possible only when we reduce activities; the fewer our actions, the greater our results. Mental chanting requires less external effort, bringing us closer to an actionless state with fewer mental activities, so we may enjoy greater results.

VRATA: SELF-DISCIPLINE

Vrata is a form of *self-discipline* in which the practitioner makes a decision to take an oath for a certain period of time. This oath becomes her spiritual practice, or sādhana. There is no external force; the practitioner takes the oath volunarily. Vrata has many benefits. It develops self-confidence, helps in conquering the senses, and fosters detachment. The practitioner performs this practice with the intention of solving some of her problems and to prepare herself for Liberation.

One form of vrata relates to food. The practitioner may decide not to eat a particular food for a period of time. For example, she may decide to eat no spices, cooked food, or food prepared by others for three years. Or she may take an oath to fast for a whole day once a week. This is different from mitāhāra and tapas because the *intention* will be different. The intention behind vrata is aimed at staying true to one's oath, or commitment.

A practitioner may also use worship as a way to develop vrata. He may take an oath to recite a particular chant, or prayer, a certain number of times each day. Or he may decide to visit a particular temple or sage every week on a particular day.

A practitioner may make a decision to sit in silence for three months. As social beings, it is very difficult for most of us to sit in silence, even for a short length of time. Isolation is very uncomfortable for the common person. Typically, one might spend one or two days in silence at most and then start feeling agitated or even a type of sadness. Thus, this type of vrata is considered a very intense practice.

These are just a few examples of how practitioners might practice this sub-limb of Aṣṭāṅga Yoga.

SIDDHĀNTA ŚRAVAṆA: LISTENING TO THE TRUTH

The last niyama is *siddhānta śravaṇa*. The goal of this practice is to try to hear only what is truthful in this universe. A practitioner will aim to restrict what he hears to only that which is true. This may relate to the ultimate Truth, or it may relate to relative truths; but the practitioner vows to hear no falsehoods. This is similar to the practice of svādhyāya in that it is an intellectual, rational approach toward learning what is necessary from one who knows. While svādhyāya, or study of the Self, focuses on a practitioner's effort to gain knowledge and understanding, siddhānta śravaṇa restricts what we hear from others.

TRUTH

The two types of truth, as we have discussed, are ultimate Truth and relative truth. Relative truth contains the knowledge that enables us to live properly in this world while proceeding toward the ultimate Truth. At the same time, we need to understand as much as possible about the ultimate Truth. To do that, we need to be as receptive as possible to the wisdom of others. We may not grasp that wisdom fully, but what we understand will give our mind a clear target. In this way, we will eliminate distractions. To accomplish this, we must practice svādhyāya, or study of the Self, as well as listen to sacred teachings in the practice of siddhānta śravaṇa.

MISCONCEPTIONS

When traveling the yogic path, many people are impeded by misconceptions about the universe, the mind and body, and the Self. Yogic techniques will not fully support us in moving toward the Eternal Truth unless we eliminate these misconceptions. Siddhānta śravaṇa helps us to do this.

Even what we know to be true may become threatened when we expose ourselves to false information. This is why it is important to limit what we hear. Many people will read the newspaper or watch television as a form of entertainment, thinking this is harmless. However, over time, the information they receive causes much harm by taking up valuable space in their mind. It can also cause them to doubt the inherent truth they already hold.

For instance, when a person has a misconceptions about milk, she may find it difficult to digest. She might think that the lactose is disturbing to her system, or that milk causes too much phlegm. Perhaps after drinking it, she even feels cramping in her stomach. While some of these reactions may be due to how dairy is being produced today, her physiology may also be refusing the benefits of milk because of her misconceptions. Individuals need to be enlightened about the true nature of milk, and then their systems will easily receive its benefits.

When we limit our exposure to false ideas, or replace them with accurate information, we gain benefits from yoga practice easily. When the student hears the Truth over and over again, he gradually becomes convinced that Realization and Liberation should be the goal of each human being's life. When that decision is firmly established, he will not deviate from this goal. That is the primary benefit of this niyama.

FIRST IMPRESSIONS

When a young aspirant first begins learning from her teacher, she will primarily hear the words of sacred texts. This listening in itself will greatly support her on her path. If her mind is unconditioned, the information can go straight to her heart and she may not need to listen for very long. However, if she is somewhat older and has previously been exposed to a lot of misinformation, then she must hear the Truth repeated often and for a longer period of time. What a seeker first hears is recorded most firmly in her mind and cannot be erased easily. If that information is wrong, it can be a severe stumbling block for any seeker. Rather than receive incorrect information, it is better to delay the start of a spiritual path until the right teacher can be found. The essential requirement is to receive correct information. In this sense, it is not a problem to wait even twenty years to find a competent teacher. If a student has refrained from hearing too many false teachings up to that point, a true teacher's transmission will quickly and easily solve the seeker's problems.

The correct interpretation of yogic philosophy is possible only if we find a Realized teacher, his direct disciple, or a sattvic person fully committed to Realization. If we are unwilling to wait for this kind of teacher, and instead collect information indiscriminately from random sources, we risk significant damage to our mind. No matter the extent of correction, the first impression is the deepest one. Because of the erroneous information we have collected, we may become unfit for yogic practice for a time, or even altogether.

When we are fully convinced of the possibility of realizing the Self, when our target is Realization and only Realization, and when we have eliminated irrelevant obstacles, we will be well on our way to the final goal. After we have become fully convinced, erroneous thoughts will gradually be eliminated. It will become very difficult to stray from our course. Grasping what a true teacher says constitutes siddhānta śravaṇa. This will fully support us on our journey toward Realization and Liberation. When we are on the right path, we will eventually achieve yogic states. This is the great benefit of siddhānta śravaṇa.

CONCLUSION: YAMAS AND NIYAMAS

Though we have discussed the yamas and niyamas in some detail, this is by no means an exhaustive study. It is simply a guide. If we wish to learn how to prepare a delicious dish to eat, it is generally not enough to read cookbooks. Better we spend some time preparing food in a kitchen with an experienced cook. In the same way, these disciplines can only be fully understood through repeated practice. Theory alone is not enough. With practice, one will develop confidence, and one's knowledge will become well established.

In order to plant a field of grain, the soil should be plowed, the weeds eliminated, and some water and perhaps fertilizer added to the ground. Finally, a fence may be built to protect the young plants. This should all occur either naturally or be deliberately tended to by a farmer. Without this kind of preparation, a field will not produce much grain. In the same way, the yamas and niyamas are essential prerequisites to begin practicing the other limbs of Aṣṭāṅga Yoga such as āsana, prāṇāyāma, pratyāhāra, and so on. The greater one's preparation, the easier the journey will be and the better the various yogic limbs of Aṣṭāṅga Yoga will become integrated. If a practitioner follows the yamas and niyamas to the maximum extent, and with an open heart, she will develop confidence on her path and gradually move firmly toward the final goal.

PART THREE

THE YOGA JOURNEY

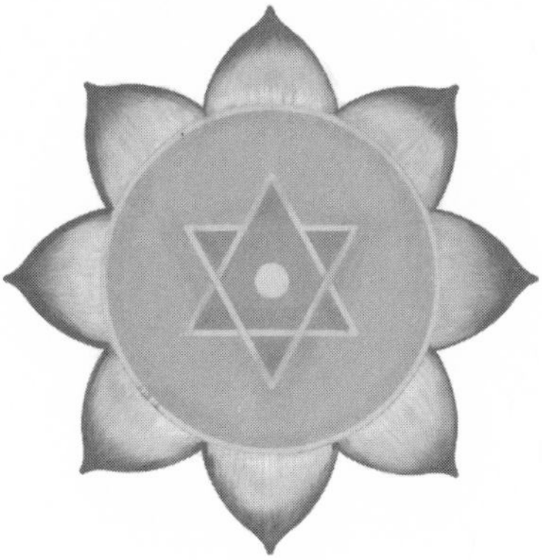

CHAPTER NINE

THE ROLE OF THE TEACHER

गुरुः साक्षत् परं ब्रह्म

IF WE WANT to understand how our body works on a physical level, we might consult a health practitioner, dietician, or even a biologist. Such a person could impart useful information, and we should take advantage of the knowledge she could offer us. It would be a waste of time, and possibly dangerous, to experiment on our body to determine whether the experts are correct. We see by their credentials and training that they have proper experience in their fields. Therefore, we trust in their advice.

Similarly, if we have questions about our taxes, we consult a tax accountant. We explain our situation, and the accountant advises us on which forms to fill out, whether to incorporate, how we might deduct business purchases, and so on. Rather than read countless books on tax regulations, we simply take this person's advice.

We should do the same thing when it comes to yoga. As yoga aspirants, we may not be able to choose the right path for ourselves. However, if we are blessed with a sincere, full-hearted quest for knowledge, we will be led to the right person. When a yogi is available to offer guidance, it is best to take his advice. Having traveled the yogic path before us, yogis have invaluable information and advice that can make the journey easier. We should recognize our good fortune in having met such a noble person and adhere to his guidance. We will gain confidence in his teachings as we use the results of our own experience to verify them.

The connection to a Realized yogi is by far the most effective way to achieve Realization. We learn through her words, her life, and, if we are fortunate, her silence. We should understand that a Realized person is the ideal representative of Nature. She is the very crown of Nature. When she is available, it is best to stay near her rather than searching elsewhere. If we are able to live nearby, a supreme, positive impact or transmission may occur naturally, allowing us to find a connection to our true Self, and thereby become Realized. This is why the role of the Realized teacher is so significant and to be treasured.

YOGIC EDUCATION

Parents play the primary role in their children learning a language. They do so not by directly teaching the child, but rather through talking to the child and to each other. As the parents move through their daily activities, the child watches, listens, and gradually learns to talk. After the child has reached a certain level of proficiency, the parents may begin to offer corrections, but primarily the education is imparted by simply being with the child, who watches and listens. That is enough. The child will learn to speak.

In a similar way, if there is an opportunity to have some connection to a Realized yogi, many things will be learned naturally. This is the most expedient path. Previously in India, this was the only method used to teach yoga. Most householders were more or less on the yogic path. Their young children were taught naturally in this manner. Older students would go to live in an āśrama to study one of the sixty-four Indian sciences. Each of these sciences would naturally prepare those students for yogic life.

Ancient texts of India reveal that this method of education was widespread. Typically, students lived in an āśrama for ten to fifteen years. Only on rare occasions would a student be directly initiated into the teachings. More often, an internal yogic atmosphere simply permeated the students' lives as they learned their external subjects. Even in the absence of direct teachings, many yogis emerged. The students realized the Eternal Truth as a matter of course.

Yogic education is based on observing and integrating the principles of Nature. It inherently gives rise to right thoughts and actions. The mind functions better and better as it becomes sharp and accurate. While this brightness and clarity help the mind function externally, they also help the mind relax. At the proper times for meditation, activity in the mind stops completely. This is yoga.

Today education tends to provoke more and more thoughts and cause various disturbances. There is no provision for true relaxation of the mind. Students are taught many unnecessary subjects, while what is most needed is absent from the curriculum. Such an approach to education does not lead to inner calmness and quietness, much less to Realization and Liberation. "Peace" is not found on the list of objectives or mission statements in most schools. An education of real value should develop the inner life of the child, the capacity to meditate, and the potential to become Realized. A competent teacher plays an integral role in this process of authentic education.

When we meet a happy and content person, we feel relaxed and happy in his presence. We feel refreshed and forget our problems. In contrast, if we meet someone who always wears a sad face and is perpetually worried, we feel the negative impact. We too may start feeling depressed. Likewise, if we spend much time with a dull person who overindulges in alcohol, we risk losing our own motivation. If we meet a learned, inspiring person, we tend to feel inspired. Simply put, we tend to emulate those around us.

There is no other material or object that affects us as much as another human being. And among human beings, the one who can influence us the most is a Realized Soul. She can kindle the spark of divine desire in our hearts, coaxing that spark into a flame. She can push us, pull us, educate us, guide us, and even carry us to our goal. She can offer the supreme guidance to experience Samādhi. There is no other method that compares to our teacher's compassion and guidance when it comes to achieving such a great goal as Realization.

A YOGI SITS IN SAMĀDHI

The mind is like a lake. It has the potential to be either very still or disturbed and muddied by waves and sediment. Ignorance, egotism, attachment, aversion, and so on are like mud in this lake of our mind, and our thoughts are like waves. Right knowledge, right companions, and right actions allow the mud to settle to the bottom. Yogic practices help us to reduce or stop the waves for a little while each day; as we begin to tame the mind, naturally the waves will subside. Our mind will become crystal clear, and if we are patient for the right opportunity, we will see an undistorted image of our true Self through this lens of the mind. At the beginning of the Rāmāyaṇa, the great ṛṣi Vālmīki prepares to bathe in the River Tamasa. As he approaches the river, he exclaims to his disciple, Bharadvāja, "Oh, how beautiful the water is. It is like the mind of a *Realized soul.*"

When a yogi sits in Samādhi, he is enjoying vastness inside himself. Because of this inner bliss, the entire state of his body changes. His posture, expression, and even the color and texture of his skin are affected. There is also an emission of energy from his body to the external world. These are common signs revealed by all yogis. Like a person who speaks with a mint in his mouth, all those around him will be affected. He may not intend for the fragrance to escape, but it will waft all around him. In this way a yogi will influence others. Even though he may be sitting absolutely motionless, he will influence everyone around him.

There are extraordinary yogis who may enter into other states besides motionless Samādhi. For example, one may open her eyes and look here and there. She may hear, touch, taste, smell, talk, and even walk. But she will not have full awareness of her body or surroundings. Her awareness may be minimal or nonexistent. She will behave somewhat like a person in the waking state, but she is not awake. In such a state, she will be known as an *avadhūta*. The great sage Śuka is an example of an avadhūta. Through all of his activities, he created a link between this world and the Divine.

THE INFLUENCE OF YOGIS

Sometimes a yogi is used as a tool of the Divine to spread Its influence. The yogi's energy is like a powerful wind carrying the fragrance of thousands of jasmine flowers. His body and mind become a medium to convey something truly remarkable to the universe. The vast energy that flows through him benefits everyone around him and, in fact, everyone in the world. If we have the help and influence of such a person, we will be directed toward the path of Liberation.

When a yoga practitioner lives around a Realized Soul, the influence of that person provides many benefits. The practitioner will automatically have correct thoughts about the type of food to eat, the type of activities to engage in, and the way to keep relationships happy and balanced. Practitioners also may get internal guidance for their yogic practice, so that they can quickly make internal progress. This help is most effective if our mind is kept calm and quiet.

The very existence of a Realized Soul indirectly supports right thinking. For instance, we may be in our car on our way to a vacation. While traveling, we may notice a place and decide to suddenly stop and stay awhile. A thought arrives: "Oh, this is a very fine place. Why don't we stay here for one day?" While we are there, we may encounter a Realized person or some other wonderful phenomenon. In this case, it is the Realized person's very presence that allows us the capacity to stop and that guides us in the direction of such an encounter. This type of correct thinking and responding actually helps solve many problems. If we are paying close attention, we realize these are significant experiences.

Residing near a Realized Soul will help release unhealthy attachments. Then, in some cases, not much practice is required to become Liberated. Given that the very purpose of practice is to correct our system, all actions taken near a Realized person will serve this purpose. Providing we have a sincere desire for Liberation, whatever right activities we undertake in her proximity become the practice itself. At some point, her presence will lead us to sit quietly and release our attachments, and we may become Realized.

At times, a Realized being may talk, other times he may be silent. His activities are not the key. He need not teach us anything. Our thinking process will change, and our attachments will be released, simply due to his presence. Many sādhakas at Ramana Maharshi's āśrama at Arunachala in Southern India had this experience. Ramana Maharshi did not implement much formal teaching. He would sometimes say a few words or sentences, but he did not spend an undue amount of time talking to his disciples. Instead, he demonstrated his love for all living beings. A few disciples would live there in his presence, eating whatever food the āśrama prepared, and spending time with him. Sometimes just sitting in his presence, meditation happened spontaneously. After a few years, a number of his disciples Realized the Eternal Truth. Such is the influence of a Realized Soul.

ROLE OF THE STUDENT

What is the role of the student? What are qualities a student should possess in order to receive Nature's grace through her teacher?

An ideal student is humble and has a thirst for knowledge. He is honest in both his words and deeds. He is straightforward, obedient, and ready to adopt an ideal yogic way of life. One notable word used to refer to an ideal student is *śiṣya,* meaning a student who embraces his teacher through his heart and allows himself to become one with his teacher; thus, a commitment develops between teacher and student that will remain true to Realization. These are just a few of the noble qualities required to receive the grace of a true teacher.

Until a teacher indicates that her teaching is complete, the student should remain dedicated. If it is not possible to physically remain in the teacher's presence, the student should remain in her presence through his heart. This commitment itself is the link whereby transmission takes place. At the end of his education, it is the student's duty to offer gurudakṣiṇā, inquiring if there is anything the teacher requires. In most cases, the teacher will not expect anything. All knowledge is sacred. It should never be sold for profit or given to an unworthy student.

Today this tradition remains to some extent in small villages here and there, but most education is becoming overly commercialized. Because of this, many who are worthy are deprived of education simply because they are poor. At the same time, those who are unworthy but wealthy easily purchase their education. As a result, knowledge is no longer transmitted in the most optimal manner. It would be better to develop a practice that takes into consideration the welfare of all humankind equally.

Also, most teachers today are only capable of guiding a portion of a student's education. In such a case, the teacher should readily lead his student to the next teacher. He should not hold on to her. At the same time, a student should never forget her honor and gratitude for her teacher. It is this gratitude that links the student to the Divine.

A train may have many boxcars. One is linked with the engine, another linked to that one, and so on down the line. When the engine moves, all the cars will move, one following the other. In this way, each is directly linked to the engine. Where the engine goes, each boxcar will go.

In the same way, there should be a connection through one's learning to the Eternal Teacher. A teacher should be the medium, not the target. A student should focus on the Divine through his teacher. There may be many teachers in between, but if there is a link to the Eternal Teacher, true learning can occur.

SEARCHING FOR A TEACHER

A student may spend years searching for a teacher, but once she finds that person, she should remain committed. Shopping from teacher to teacher easily spoils the heart connection required to develop a meaningful teacher-student relationship. When there are multiple influences, a student develops a confusing mix of impressions that can have a negative impact.

TEACHING WHAT YOU HAVE LEARNED

In some cases, the teacher will come to expect the student to convey his knowledge to other worthy students. But it is the teacher alone who should decide this. Not all who are taught are capable of teaching others. Even if one may have some knowledge and skills to teach, it should be reserved for those who are well established in divine qualities. Only students established in noble qualities should be considered teachers, because the qualities of the teacher get transmitted to the students.

If a student does not receive permission from her teacher, begins teaching, and fails to acknowledge the proper source of her own teaching, that becomes a form of stealing. Moreover, a student will not acquire proper knowledge, or the skills to teach such knowledge, without the permission and grace of her teacher. Although a Realized person is the ideal teacher, a Realized person may not be easy to find, in which case, only those who are humble and devoted to Realization should be selected as teachers.

THE INNER TEACHER

When peering into a lake, we will not see the reflection of our face if the water is muddy and choppy. But if the mud settles to the bottom, and the wind is naturally still, we can easily see our own undistorted reflection. In the same way, if we want to see who we really are, we must still the mind. If the major influences in our life are consumerism, money, and extravagant materials, we will have a vast number of incorrect thoughts and other problems. If the major influence is a Realized Soul, our mind will be calm and quiet. We will receive right thoughts, and this will solve many problems. Right thinking is a key benefit of being associated with a Realized Soul.

It may be impossible for us to think correctly all the time. We receive certain thoughts according to our karma, from which we cannot completely escape. These thoughts may be positive or negative and cause both joyous and sorrowful experiences.

Simultaneously, our mind has the capacity to receive thoughts according to our intention. These thoughts, too, may be positive or negative, but if we work to cultivate a calm and quiet mind, we will receive more positive thoughts. Maintaining a well-balanced mind and body, and having a connection with a Realized Soul, fosters correct thinking. However, because of so many imbalances found in our society today, we have lost much of our capacity for right thinking. Hence, we find more problems than solutions in our thinking. When our mind is disturbed, we cannot distinguish right thoughts from those caused by our undesirable karmas and saṃskāras.

Yoga practitioners sometimes pray for the right thoughts above all else. There is a proverb in India that explains, "If you pray to the gods and goddesses for support, they will not appear to you in a physical form but will prompt you with correct thoughts."

Correct thoughts, and the actions that we undertake based on those thoughts, eliminate our miseries. We receive the most genuine spiritual help internally, not externally. If our thinking is clear and accurate, we will receive all possible types of support for our spiritual and physical welfare. If we have errors in our thought process, then our welfare at all levels will be at risk.

We might pray for help with some financial problems. What type of support can the gods and goddesses give us? They cannot arrive in human form with a checkbook. But they can give us correct thoughts. We might understand that we have a compulsion to spend money in a certain area, and we might learn how to stop that bad habit. We might have an insight about an honorable new way to earn money. We might have a better view about the correct use of money.

If a piece of wood covered in a thick layer of clay is thrown into water, it will sink. But gradually, as the clay or mud dissolves, the wood will rise to the surface. No effort is required to achieve this. In a similar way, the mind is not able to enjoy the Eternal Truth because it is bound to the external world by attachments. For example, we might find ourselves attached to our wife or husband, friends, or other family members. Other common hooks are our body, home, job, money, prestige, fame, and worldly accomplishments. These hooks drag our minds to the external world. If we eliminate these attachments, the very nature of the mind withdraws inwardly. Having a husband or wife, a house, or a job is not intrinsically contrary to yogic practice, but if we are overly attached, this will impede our inward journey.

ADVICE FROM THE SAGES

Sages advise that the first step is to precisely determine our goal. Next, we should sincerely and strongly crave this goal. Furthermore, they recommend that we become fully absorbed in some particular *vehicle* that will help carry us to our goal. For example, if we contemplate and meditate fully on a Realized Soul, on her image or photograph, a transformation gradually takes place. Based on the influence of that yogi and certain characteristics of her image, we can realize the Eternal Truth.

This is not as strange as it may seem. We are influenced by many things in this world, from where we live to the weather and the food we eat. Even the clothes we wear affect us. However, it is the people around us that make the greatest impression.

For example, our parents strongly influence us from a very early age. We watch and imitate them over many years. We are also influenced by friends and peers. Throughout life there are countless examples of profound impressions made by the people around us. We are shaped more by human beings than anything else in the universe. But among human beings, whose influence will be felt most strongly? Who has the highest capacity to change the way we think? Who can thoroughly educate us regarding the purpose of this human life? Who can provide the best model for us to emulate? Only one who is Realized. He will become our Eternal Teacher, who can guide us like no one else.

Our physical location does not matter, whether we are in India, the United States, Europe, or somewhere else. Thoughts can travel anywhere in the universe. If we have close connections with a yogi, we will gravitate to her presence, either in this birth or another. The influence of the yogi will eventually solve all of our problems, so that we can become Liberated. But in order for this to transpire, we need to have some kind of attachment to yogic ideals. We need to redirect our attachment to a yogi, or to her teachings, behavior, character, or even external appearance. Anything related to her can support our quest for Liberation. Any material in the universe can support Liberation, but something related to a Liberated Soul will have the greatest possible influence.

INTUITION

If there is a flood, we will look for a boat to take us to safe, dry land. If there is no boat, we must try to swim. These are examples of *human effort.* In addition to human effort, we may get support from Nature, or the Divine. Patañjali says that the all-pervading Eternal Truth is itself the teacher of all teachers. One may find guidance through external nature, or one may find guidance from within. This is a kind of intuition that comes to us through the grace of the Eternal Truth—the Teacher of all teachers.

But this kind of intuition may work only when there is no alternative to guide us. For example, imagine that a person who lives in a very remote region gets sick and has no chance of reaching a doctor for help. In such a desperate situation, this person's intuition will begin to guide him as to how to take care of himself. However, if a doctor happens to be within reach, the patient's intuition will not work as powerfully. Even if he attempts to call on this inner voice, his system may not fully cooperate, and he might even arrive at the wrong intuition. Thus, for inevitable situations, Nature gives us inner resources and acts to guide us. But this should not be misunderstood and misused. The Divine expects us to use our human effort.

When there is no Realized person to guide us, we must try by ourselves—but only as a last resort. Nature wants everyone to realize the Self. She is constantly offering us help to move in that direction. This is the grace of Nature, or God, and it exists everywhere and at all times. The human mind, as a tool of Nature, is capable of solving any problem, providing it is used correctly. Through the use of our mind and body, and with sincere effort, it is possible to progress on a correctly chosen yogic path. No one is ever deprived of this opportunity. This is true whether you are rich or poor, man or woman, young or old, rational or emotional, educated or uneducated, Western or Indian: A yogic path is available to all. However, just as it is best to consult a knowledgeable physician when we are unhealthy, a yogic path is best navigated with the help of a Realized teacher.

GRACE OF THE ETERNAL TEACHER

As a young man in the early 1970s, I studied Saṃskṛta at the Saṃskṛta College of Mysore. This is also where I studied many of the classical texts on yoga under the guidance of gifted Saṃskṛta scholars. As I went through these texts multiple times, I developed confidence in my understanding of yoga.

At the same time, I began to follow many disciplines and practices outlined by the yamas and niyamas. I began to notice many changes in my body. I became slim, light, and very flexible. My digestion was excellent, I was able to function on comparatively little sleep, and my memory became very keen. Gradually, I noticed more subtle changes in my system, including various yogic achievements. Though these were very minor achievements, they helped develop a confidence within me. Slowly, I began to understand the powerful nature of these yogic practices.

As I advanced in my prāṇāyāma and meditation practice, I began to experience leaving my body and moving through space with the subtle mind. While this was very pleasurable, it also frightened me. At times

I even had the feeling that I would be unable to return to my body. At a certain period, this fear arose each time I began my practice. I soon realized that it was a fear of death itself.

I began to search for information about these experiences in the ancient yogic texts and elsewhere. I talked with various people whom I thought might be familiar with these phenomena but did not receive any practical answers. At one point, I even traveled three days by train to Haridwar and Hrushikesh; I met and talked with many people but still found no satisfactory answers—though I simply may have missed meeting the right person at that time.

In desperation, I decided to try and meet the renowned Monk of Kañcikāmakoṭipīṭha, Śrī Śrī Chandra Shekhara Sarasvatī. He was known to be well established on the yogic path and firmly committed to the goal of Realization. I had heard this monk was staying in a cowshed at a Brahmin's home some twenty kilometers away from Kañci. One of my best friends, who shared an intense interest in yoga and Realization, also wished to meet this monk. One full moon night, we decided to walk to the remote village to visit him.

We arrived at 3 A.M. We spoke with an attendant outside the house and expressed our desire to speak with their *swamiji*. Suddenly, from behind the gate, we heard the monk call for us. We were then led to the cowshed. We saluted the monk, and I began to explain in Saṃskṛta why I had come.

I spoke about my experience and fears. He listened silently. Then he closed his eyes and went into a deep trance. At least ten or fifteen minutes passed before he opened his eyes and said, "Do not worry. You are on the right path. Simply contemplate on the all-pervading Great Light, *Brahma*. Now go back." He then blessed us, offering us auspicious yellow rice and fruits.

As I arrived back at Mysore, one of my favorite and honorable teachers, Śrī Sheshachla Sharma, asked why I had been absent from school. At first, I was reluctant to tell him the truth, but he persisted in asking. Finally, I revealed to him the concerns I had about my practice and my meeting the Monk of Kañci. He listened with great compassion. Then, by the grace of the Eternal Truth, he began to tell me about his Eternal Teacher, the great yogi Śrī Raṅga. Thus, on that day, I was led to the very person who would become my guide and Eternal Teacher for the rest of my life!

From my grandmother teaching me Saṃskṛta chants early in the morning along the Tunga River to my Saṃskṛta teacher's advice, to my fateful decision to board the Mysore bus against my father's wish, to my honorable teacher's inquiry as to my absence from school—all of these incidents were the favorable winds that guided me to discover a true yogic path. Like a spinning coin before it settles, events turned me here and there before I found a place to rest. I have always felt grateful for this series of events—and play of the Divine—that brought me into contact with my teacher and onto a final path.

SILENCE, THE GREAT TEACHER

Shankaracharya, the great philosopher of nondualism, was also a poet. In one poem, he narrated the following incident:

A few elderly people wished to receive lessons on Liberation from a Realized teacher. They traveled far from their homes in order to meet a highly respected man. They arrived expecting to find an elderly person who would answer all their questions, but to their surprise, they discovered a mere youth sitting under a banyan tree. These elderly people were anxious to receive answers to their questions: What is the Eternal Truth? How can we experience it? Who are we? What is the right path for us? But the youth did not attempt to answer, or even speak to them. Instead, he sat cross-legged on the ground in *padmāsana,* "lotus posture," closed his eyes, and went into a deep meditation.

At first, the elderly people did not understand. But soon they, too, began to sit down and enter into meditation. After some time, the hairs on their arms suddenly stood on end, and their hearts were touched to the deepest core. These elderly people were moved to tears and overwhelmed with gratitude toward their young teacher. They bowed to him, sharing words of gratitude, "We came here troubled by many questions, but they have all been answered. We feel content and may now return to our homes."

Shankaracharya reflected that this incident presented a marvelous wonder: All the youth did was simply sit in silence, and the elderly persons' questions were all answered. This was a yogic experience; the youth was in Samādhi.

This story can also be seen as a metaphor. The "elderly" symbolize those who are disturbed by the materialistic world; the "youth," having taken refuge in his yogic bliss, remains in his original, undisturbed condition. The chronological age of a Realized person is irrelevant. He might be fifteen years old, or he might be seventy. The questions the elders ask represent a quest of the heart, not of the tongue. The answers came not through words but through an experience. For such questions, mere speech is a poor medium; silence is the best educator. The hairs on the elders' arms stood on end as a sign of their experience of the Eternal Truth. They discovered their true home to be in their hearts.

The great sage and my Honorable Teacher, Śrī Raṅga, said, "This external world is like a rented house. It does not really belong to us. It is impermanent. However, you have the right to move into a permanent mansion. This is the abode of Eternal Happiness. So finish your duties as quickly as possible and strive to attain that which is your birthright. Go now and occupy your true home, which is inside of you."

CHAPTER TEN

THE MANGO ORCHARD

एकं लक्ष्यम्

THERE ONCE WAS a small village within a vast kingdom that possessed a few ordinary mango orchards. The villagers enjoyed these trees very much, but they heard rumors about a more wonderful mango grove situated within the king's preserve. Apparently, the mangos in that orchard were incomparably sweet and fragrant and unlike any other mangos seen in the kingdom. However, no one in the village had ever seen this orchard. Not only was it difficult to receive permission to visit, but the orchard was located in a distant mountainous region. Moreover, the road there was very difficult to travel.

For many years the orchard was closed to the public. Then one day, the manager of the king's preserve announced that he was granting permission for a few people to travel within its borders. There was one stipulation: No one would be allowed to spend the night.

Soon a group of villagers got together and made a heartfelt request to visit the prized orchard. The king's ministers heard their request and granted permission. Quickly, the group began preparations for their journey. Together, they represented a cross-section of the village's residents, including a doctor, a chemist, an engineer, a farmer, an accountant, and a common man who had no special training or education. Everyone in the group had heard about this legendary mango orchard and was very eager to see and enjoy it firsthand.

As agreed, the villagers arranged to complete the entire trip within one day. They planned the trip to fall on the full moon, so that they could start before daylight. They estimated that if they left very early, they could reach the mango orchard by noon. Then, before returning, they might fully enjoy a few hours within the grove before sundown.

When the group embarked upon their journey, they encountered many obstacles, including a lake they had to cross by boat, a large river they had to ford, and a mountainous region inhabited by bears, mountain lions, and many other wild animals. After the sun rose, there was a long stretch with no water during the heat of the day. With much effort, the travelers overcame all these obstacles safely and arrived at the mango orchard by midday. In their anticipation to see the orchard, they forgot how hungry and thirsty they were.

One by one, each member of the group began to examine the mango orchard according to his own interest. The doctor focused on the tree's medicinal properties. He wondered whether the leaves might eliminate certain disorders. He wondered whether the shadow of the mango trees provoked pitta or vāta. He studied the trees' bark and the possible medicinal uses of their roots.

The chemist investigated the minerals that were present in the soil, postulating that the chemical makeup of the land was responsible for producing such delicious mangos. He wondered which nutrients might be responsible for the beautiful color of the mangos' skin. Further, he analyzed the chemical compositions of the trees' bark, wood, and roots.

The engineer was in awe of the size of the mangos, and he marveled that the trees were even able to stand. He immediately began calculating the weight of the fruit-laden branches and the size and reach of the root systems. He estimated the effect of wind on the trees and pondered what might happen in the event of a huge storm.

The farmer was impressed with the fertility of the land. He wondered how much rainfall this orchard might require and how the water table might affect the orchard. He wondered how much time it would take to grow such an orchard and how much farming it would require.

The accountant at once began counting the mangos in each tree. He calculated the expense of growing such trees, figuring in the human effort, the money for seed, the cost of acquiring the land, and so on. He also computed the enormous profits to be made by such an orchard.

In contrast to these professionals, the common man had no intention other than to enjoy the mangos and to satisfy his hunger and thirst. When he arrived at the orchard, he was hot and tired, so he climbed a tree, picked some mangos, and sat in the shade to eat them. He felt very happy and content simply sitting and eating his mangos. They were perfectly ripe, exceptionally tasty, and wonderfully satisfying. He felt that the mangos and the orchard were marvelous, and he was so happy that he forgot the whole world. He could not even compare his happiness with any that he had felt previously in the village, or with what he had experienced eating any other types of fruit or food. He also thoroughly enjoyed the peaceful atmosphere of the orchard. Because of his intense pleasure, he sat quietly, appreciating the grace of Nature. He humbly expressed his gratitude to God for creating the universe. In return, he felt even more peace and calm. Unknowingly, he fell into a deep meditation on God, and, because of his calmness and quietness, he felt God's presence within him.

Evening came, and the group had to quickly prepare to leave and return to their village. To their great disappointment, the scientists and other professionals suddenly realized that they had completely forgotten to eat any mangos or to simply enjoy the atmosphere of the orchard. Only the common man had experienced these pleasures.

In a similar way, because of our saṃskāra, habits, and interests, we may easily forget the most important thing in life. Our human body is like a mango tree that can provide us with wonderful fruit. This fruit comes in the form of peace, calm, quiet, contentment, and an unimaginable bliss. Yet we can enjoy this fruit only when we fix our attention firmly on the right goal and forget our extensive preoccupation with the external world. We need not be obsessed with deep investigations and inquiry; like the common man, we can simply climb the tree, pick the mangos, and enjoy them.

We have been longing for a human birth for a very long time. When we use our human body as it was intended, we have the capacity to enjoy these wonderful results. Because of our forgetfulness, we have developed interests that distract us from our primary goal. We might spend our whole life pursuing these distractions. Then, at the end of our time, just like the professionals in the story, we tragically realize that we have wasted a precious opportunity. We may repent, but it will be too late. We will be in the twilight of our lives, and we will have to leave the orchard. We will have lost our chance, and we will need to take another birth. This is the pattern of most human lives. The tragedy of the human condition is that we forget, again and again, about the incomparable happiness that could be ours.

Because of this, yogis recommend that we do not spend too much time attempting to understand the universe. Certainly, we must gain some essential knowledge, but even while doing so, we must commence our journey toward the Eternal Truth. The most important thing to know is what is essential for contemplation of the Soul and for Liberation. It is best we study that which is nearest to us, our Self. The Self is within our reach. This study is one that we can complete and that will yield more fruit than any other possible study of the external world.

Even while we are studying yoga and the Self, we need to limit the tendency to explore every subject to the utmost detail. Each yama and niyama works according to certain principles. It is possible to spend our entire life researching the dynamics and mechanisms behind any one of them. It is useful to have some basic understanding about their importance and how our system responds to these practices, but it is better not to spend our entire lives attempting a full investigation. Mere rational thought processes will not lead us to correct conclusions, much less to the final goal.

The rational approach that most people take in today's world has led to the misunderstanding of many hidden truths; the result of this is widespread confusion. This external world is managed by the Divine world. Thus, we can understand much of the external world in depth only through yogic sight, which is intended for this purpose. If we are able to accept some of the yogic principles with trust and faith, and spend most of our time practicing to quiet our minds, we will be able to enjoy the bliss of our own "mango tree." This, after all, is our foremost goal.

I wish to add emphasis here, because minds that are extroverted by nature will tend to be extroverted in all activities. If we take a monkey to a calm and quiet place, it will not hesitate to cause disturbances and mischief. Rather than the quietness of a place influencing the monkey, the monkey will inflict its disturbing nature wherever it goes. Similarly, when we bring a noisy mind to the science of quietness, the mind will be noisy in its investigations of that quietness. Until we gain some skill, we will lose the most important benefit, calmness and quietness.

If we want to enjoy a deep sleep, we need to follow some basic principles of health, rather than engaging in an intense study of sleep itself. An average person is not interested in the science of sleep. She may not even have the capacity to immerse herself in such a study. Moreover, such a study would require years to complete. Yet, we all need sleep. Even a medical doctor who has specialized in the study of sleep needs to follow a few basic principles when it is time for her to rest. At bedtime, she must forget all her knowledge, lie on her bed in a quiet, darkened room, and enjoy her sleep. If she constantly thinks about the mechanics of sleep while trying to go to sleep, her knowledge about sleep will itself be a hindrance to sleeping. In this way, information about sleep, though true, may spoil our capacity to fall asleep.

Normally, we spend our time involved in worldly affairs. This is primarily how we use our mind. But there is something wonderful to uncover within the mind itself. We spend so much time trying to understand the external world, yet we rarely look intensely at what is closest to us—our own mind and body. If we forget about worldly affairs and try to find the Eternal Light abiding within us, then, as our focus intensifies, we will visualize it.

A common man is in need of yogic bliss. This bliss is possible to attain through practicing certain disciplines. Whether we fully understand how or why a particular practice works, if we follow these practices, we will experience that bliss. If we do not follow these disciplines, we will not be able to enjoy this bliss, no matter how much we know about yogic technique. The Upaniṣads tell us that we must first learn something about the universe and the Divine; then we must forget all that we have learned in order to fully enjoy the bliss. Though a man who is hungry for corn may purchase it with its husk, when it comes time to eat the corn, he will peel the husk from the cob and throw it away, eating only the kernels. In the same way, we must try to understand a little about the Divine. Then, at the time of our practice, we must forget all that we have learned and concentrate on our practice alone. If we want to enjoy eating a mango, we need not know everything there is to know about the biology and cultivation of the mango tree.

CHAPTER ELEVEN

CONCLUSION

शान्तिः

IN THIS BOOK, we have explored some of the basic principles of yoga. In today's world, we are all accustomed to intellectual analysis with an eye toward cause and effect. Indeed, this is a good approach; but it has its limitations, because Nature always hides things. Even though we think we have thoroughly explored some aspect of Nature, we soon come to realize that there are ever more hidden layers. Sometimes Nature makes these layers extraordinarily difficult for us to probe. In many ways, the search for external knowledge is endless. We can seek out hidden truths in the universe, but the joy and contentment that we gain from this research is limited and fleeting at best. Rather than focus exclusively on gaining knowledge about the workings of this external world, it is infinitely more rewarding to develop an intense quest of knowledge about the Self. Such knowledge brings unlimited and lasting pleasure and bliss.

This book began with the story of the prince, uprooted from his true home and guided by a Realized sage to a triumphant return to rule his father's kingdom. When he began thinking of himself as a prince, his princely qualities slowly evolved. This was possible only because these were already his natural qualities. The conception of himself as a hunter's child was only a hindrance to his natural growth. His food, thoughts, and activities were all restricted by the constraints of a hunter's life. Whether or not the prince understood the process of his growth, the growth was possible only because of his inherent princely nature.

In the same way, we, too, have this wonderful opportunity to apply practical techniques and knowledge that might enable us to regain the divine qualities inherent in us. This is our birthright as human beings. It is possible simply by trusting the guidance of a yogi, or Nature herself.

The story of the prince and the story of the mango orchard both offer us essential kernels of knowledge about our duty in this human life. If we take this to heart, we can enjoy the wonderful results of this life and ultimately be Liberated from the cycle of birth and death.

May you allow the favorable winds to guide you on your yogic journey!

APPENDIX ONE

An Overview of the Traditional Branches of Yoga

THREE LIMBS OF JÑĀNA YOGA

Jñāna Yoga possesses three limbs: *śravaṇa, manana,* and *nidhidhyāsana.* In *śravaṇa,* the student focuses on hearing direct experience and advice from a Realized Soul. If this is not possible, the student may listen to a knowledgeable person read sacred scriptures like the Upaniṣads, the Bhagavad-Gītā, and others. *Manana* refers to recollecting what one has heard or learned and deeply contemplating that until one has acquired a profound understanding of its meaning. The student must then absorb what he has heard or learned with a firm understanding. *Nīdhidyāsana* means meditating directly on the Eternal Truth, or the OṂ sound. Here the student must possess the capacity to grasp a spark of the Divine and use it as the object of his meditation.

Jñāna Yoga is also known as *Sāṅkhya Yoga*. The word *saṅkhya* means "number"; Sāṅkhya Yoga refers to a practice of deep contemplation on the twenty-four steps of evolution found in the creation of the body and the entire universe. The practitioner identifies each step concluding, "I am not this; *this is not the Soul.*" Once the practitioner goes through all components of the body, she arrives at a deep awareness of the indissoluble "I." This is how she will come to realize the Eternal Truth. All three limbs of Jñāna Yoga are used for this deep contemplation and are considered integral for this practice. Therefore, Jñāna Yoga and Sāṅkhya Yoga are often considered one and the same.

Various subpaths are linked to Jñāna Yoga. Each shares this type of deep meditation practice as its central technique. Two of these subpaths are Rāja Yoga and Laya Yoga.

RĀJA YOGA: THE KINGLY PATH

Each yogic path addresses specific imbalances in the mind and body. Some people are fortunate enough to inherently maintain balance in all aspects of life. Such an individual need not involve herself in many practices. Such a person is capable of meditating very easily without the use of techniques such as āsana, prāṇāyāma, or mudrās. Because she can start meditating directly, Rāja Yoga is the appropriate path for her. Rāja Yoga begins directly with meditation and contains only two limbs: dhyāna (meditation practice) and the practice of Samādhi.

Rāja means "king." Thus, Rāja Yoga is known as "the kingly path." All valid yoga paths converge in meditation, and meditation culminates in Samādhi. This path begins with meditation, as other practices are unnecessary—hence its regal title. A Rāja Yoga practitioner will accept certain objects for meditation. When he focuses on these objects, his mind will merge into the causal state and he will visualize the Eternal Truth. Since Rāja Yoga is a branch of Jñāna Yoga, some call this practice Jñāna Yoga.

LAYA YOGA: MERGING THE MIND

When we watch an enthralling movie or play, we gradually lose ourselves in it. We become totally involved, fully empathizing with the hero or heroine. Their problems become our problems. We may not be aware of the chair we are sitting on or hear if someone calls us. We often forget about the external world entirely, including our personal problems. Our mind becomes fully merged with the drama.

This may also occur while concentrating on an intense intellectual problem. Here, too, our awareness of external sensations decreases the more deeply we probe. As we intensely focus the mind, all external awareness begins to disappear. This is what we mean when we speak of "merging the mind." This merging is known as *laya,* and using this technique for Liberation is Laya Yoga. By following certain disciplines, the mind will be merged into its original condition, or *causal state*. The yogic text *Amanaska Yoga* is the authoritative text on Laya Yoga.

As we discussed earlier, yogic theory describes four subtle states, or stages, of the mind: manas, ahaṅkāra, mahat, and pradhāna. Manas is what is most commonly meant when referring to the mind in English. Manas merges into ahaṅkāra, where the consciousness of "I" resides. Ahaṅkāra merges into mahat, where a deity, bliss, or light may be experienced. Finally, mahat merges into pradhāna, where one finds total stillness of the mind. This leads to Realization. Laya Yoga is the process of intentionally merging the mind from stage to stage.

In this practice, the mind is kept calm and quiet while the practitioner observes this merging nature of the mind. The practitioner may watch all four of these stages constantly moving through the mind, one after another. As he carefully identifies aspects related to ahaṅkāra, the mind will automatically dissolve into ahaṅkāra. In the same way, when the mind is dissolved into ahaṅkāra, the practitioner will contemplate mahat. He will feel, "Oh, this is an aspect of mahat," and ahaṅkāra will be merged into mahat. Once established in mahat, the mind will more easily remain calm and quiet. Understanding this yogic anatomy of the mind, a practitioner can learn to merge the mind from stage to stage.

The mind is like a movie screen, in that the external world of objects is projected onto it as a movie is projected onto a screen. However, the light of the Eternal Truth also shines on the mind, waiting for our discovery. Using the analogy of the mind as a screen, these four stages are constantly being projected onto the mind. Manas appears to be the most powerful because in today's world, this is where our attention is primarily directed. As a consequence, most people are unfamiliar and inexperienced with the remaining three stages. In fact, after a practitioner learns to turn the mind inward and develops an intense longing and attraction for the internal states, she will conclude that the relative powers of the four stages are reversed. From an internal point of view, pradhāna is by far the most powerful or attractive projection, and manas the least.

Merging manas into its causal state is common in all yogic techniques; however, Laya Yoga is more deliberately focused. Keep in mind that no one path is for all practitioners. Some may find it extremely difficult to distinguish these four stages of the mind's inward movement. Of course, we all tend to be much more aware of external objects than of the occasional moments of quietness in our mind. But if we are keen observers, we can learn to detect the more subtle projections. It takes more patience than skill to observe the mind moving inward.

Unfortunately, few take the time to thoroughly examine their own mind or to distinguish and identify this movement that may naturally occur for all of us. A clever observer will learn to recognize even the faintest projection on the screen of their mind.

KARMA YOGA: A JOURNEY TO INNER LIGHT

We have already discussed how we become lost in the forest of the external world. The reason for our predicament lies within our actions, or karma. We have entered the forest, and now additional action is required to remedy our situation. Just as a knowledgeable and compassionate person can advise a lost wanderer on how to return home, the path of Karma Yoga can guide us with the right actions necessary to reach our final goal. Thus, Karma Yoga is the yoga of *right action.*

Our bodies are made for action. If we do not perform actions, we cannot exist. However, because we sometimes engage in inappropriate actions and behaviors, imbalances occur in our system. Nature will attempt to correct these errors and bring our system back into balance. If we accept Nature's corrections, we can eliminate many of our problems. But due to māyā's influence, we are often unable to fully grasp the hidden messages Nature provides. Thus, we require some guidance.

The practice of Karma Yoga requires us to understand right action and then to engage in it for an extended period of time. The key is to engage in such right action without being attached to its results. If we do this, day by day our body will come to a natural condition of health and balance. Gradually, we will gain this health because we are living according to the divine principles of Nature. When our actions are in harmony with our system, many of our previous errors are eliminated. When they are sufficiently reduced, we will have fewer thoughts and modifications of mind. Our tendency for future error will be greatly limited. This is how the practice of Karma Yoga brings a practitioner to gradually experience Samādhi.

Haṭha Yoga and Aṣṭāṅga Yoga are considered subpaths of Karma Yoga. This is because the role of human effort and action underlies their various disciplines.

HAṬHA YOGA: BODY AND BREATH AS VEHICLES

The mind and body are closely attuned to one another. There is a direct link between the two. If we adjust the mind correctly, the body moves toward balance; if we adjust the body correctly, the mind moves toward balance. Mantra Yoga, Laya Yoga, and Rāja Yoga are all yogic paths that use disciplines to adjust the *mind* so as to allow it to move inward. In contrast, Haṭha Yoga uses disciplines to adjust the *body* so as to allow the mind to move inward. With sufficient understanding and discipline, a practitioner may achieve yogic experiences and visualize the Eternal Truth. Haṭha Yoga is considered a subpath of Karma Yoga. It also functions as a ladder to Rāja Yoga in that its disciplines purify the body and build mental capacity.

Limbs of Haṭha Yoga. Haṭha Yoga primarily outlines the use of physical yogic techniques and contains four primary limbs: āsana, prāṇāyāma, mudrā, and nādānusandhana. The first limb, āsana, requires a practitioner to become well established in a comfortable and stable sitting posture. The second limb teaches disciplines aimed at breath control, or prāṇāyāma, that help the mind move inward. For example, if we pay close attention to our breath, we will discover that we are breathing with primarily the right nostril or the left nostril; moreover, this changes throughout the day as we move from one activity to the next. There are a few simple techniques to unite the breath of the right and left nostrils. As the breath moves equally between the right and left nostrils, sattva is provoked and the mind moves internally. Thus, the practitioner moves toward the yogic experience.

Haṭha Yoga's use of āsana is not the same as is generally taught in the world today. In Haṭha Yoga, there are two types of āsana: One is for elimination of toxins in order to correct the body or mind; the other is intended for meditation. Each possesses a primary function, though both may work for either purpose.

In the next limb, practitioners use certain *mudrās,* or postures formed by the hands, legs, and face. As one moves inward on the yogic journey, mudrās sometimes occur spontaneously, and a practitioner may use these postures to help deepen her practice. Finally, in *nādānusādhana* a practitioner may hear a divine sound and contemplate it.

Overall, some combination of all four Haṭha Yoga techniques can support the mind to begin its inward journey. However, there is a fifth limb offered in Haṭha Yoga known as *ṣaṭkarma,* or *ṣaṭkriya.* It consists of six cleansing techniques known as *neti, dhauti, basti, kapālabhāti, trāṭaka,* and *nauli.* This limb is an option to practice for persons having excess vāta, pitta, or kapha in their body. It is considered optional, because prāṇāyāma can also solve these problems.

In the traditional sense, *āsana* refers to a particular stable sitting posture that a practitioner holds for a long period of time without any movement or discomfort. This is āsana intended for meditation. It should lead to some experience of happiness or bliss. *Pādāṅguṣṭāsana* (hand on the big toe pose), *trikoṇāsana* (triangle pose), and *ūrdhva dhanurāsana* (back bending pose) are examples of āsanas for correcting the body. These types of āsana are not practiced for many hours at a stretch; rather, they are done only for a few minutes each when the body is in need of the specific correction they provide.

We would think it foolish to enter a pharmacy and request every medicine in the shop. We use only those medicines that are needed to correct a specific problem we might be experiencing at a given time. In the same way, it is not necessary to do many āsanas. A competent teacher should determine what corrections a practitioner needs in his mind or body and then prescribe the appropriate postures for those specific corrections. Āsanas for elimination of toxins and correction of the body should be used only until the body becomes rebalanced. After that, only meditation postures are recommended.

The *Haṭha Yoga Pradīpikā* and the *Gheraṇḍa Samhitā* are the two authoritative and authentic texts for Haṭha Yoga. The *Haṭha Yoga Pradīpika* explains a number of postures and disciplines that are useful, though in the end it recommends only four stable sitting postures: *siddhāsana, padmāsana, siṃhāsana,* and *bhadrāsana.* These are the most important āsanas of all. One of those four, siddhāsana, is the most comfortable and stable. The *Haṭha Yoga Pradīpikā* states that this posture is the "kingly" posture. If we fully master this one posture, there is actually nothing else we need to know about yoga. With such mastery, a practitioner should be able to sit for three hours or longer, without the slightest discomfort or movement. The mind will quiet, and deep meditation will be possible as a result of consistent practice of siddhāsana.

However, based on the practitioner's constitution, health, and body condition, a number of alternative āsanas may be prescribed for periods of time.

BHAKTI YOGA: THE PATH OF DEVOTION

Many people have a tendency toward deep attachment. This tendency binds them to the cycle of birth and death. Through ignorance, they become attached to some worldly object or material such as money, power, sensual pleasure, or the like. These are all powerful hooks that ensnare us and only create further cravings and attachments. Fortunately, our tendency for attachment can itself be used for Liberation. For this to occur, we must substitute for these familiar objects of attachment those associated with the Eternal Truth. This is Bhakti Yoga, the path of devotion.

As explained in a story at the beginning of the sixth chapter, we enter into a forest because of external cravings and attachments—to enjoy the beautiful views and search for flowers and precious herbs. However, we find our way home through our newly found attachment to the words and teachings of our guide. Bhakti Yoga encourages us to use attachment to find our way to the Divine, our true home. The great sages say, "Use this very attachment that has caught you to free yourself from its grip. Simply change your direction and attach yourself to some divine object that is nearer to the Eternal Truth, and it will then become your link to it."

One of the many subpaths of Bhakti Yoga is Mantra Yoga.

MANTRA YOGA: SOUND & THE EVOLUTION OF THE UNIVERSE

Practitioners of Mantra Yoga chant regularly for hours at a time. When they receive the results of their practice, they visualize the deities whose sacred mantra was taught to them by their teacher. In this tradition, there are thousands of mantras, each used for a specific purpose. The specific purpose will depend upon the role this divine energy plays in the universe. Some mantras have the goal of Liberation. Others support the practitioner in visualizing a particular deity and gaining his or her blessings or simply accessing his or her source of energy. Often, names such as Rāma and Kṛṣṇa function as mantras. Not only are they names of important and beloved *incarnations,* they are also connected with the particular centers in the body where those divine energies reside. Their names came from the original Saṃskṛta syllable combinations that invoke that particular energy in the universe.

A teacher selects a mantra for his student based on the student's constitution and saṃskāra. The student regularly chants the mantra while also maintaining other disciplines. At some point, her mind will merge into the mantra. The mantra then serves as a vehicle, and she receives the results of the mantra. Some mantras have limitations and can only carry a practitioner to a certain point. In this case, the practitioner will need to receive a new mantra to carry her farther. Then again, there are some mantras that, if chanted properly, can take the practitioner all the way to the final goal of visualizing the Eternal Truth.

As per time-honored tradition, mantras are normally given to a student through initiation. Unless there is an initiation, they are not used. Moreover, a knowledgeable teacher will only initiate a mantra to a student capable of using that mantra in a correct manner. This is, in part, due to the adverse impact a mantra may have on the teacher himself if it is not used correctly.

Following Indian tradition, female practitioners do not chant the Oṃ sound, Gāyatrī, or other Vedic mantras. This is due to specific female constitutional factors. Proper pronunciation of mantra requires *mūla bandha*—firm holding of the perineum and rectum muscles. Over a long period of time, this particular technique can disturb a woman's menstruation cycle, which can lead to various physical and psychological disturbances. It may even affect a woman's pregnancy and childbirth. In general, disciplines of intense chanting develop an upward movement in the body that conflicts with the natural flow and constitution of a woman's body.

THE KEY TO THE LIFE OF MANTRA

There are two varieties of mantras: *Vedic* mantra and *Laukika* mantra. A Vedic mantra requires precise pronunciation. It derives its power, its life, from the exact sound of the mantra. It should be given only to a practitioner who has the capacity for exact pronunciation. It should also only be given to a student who has the capacity for maintaining specific disciplines that will fully support the mantra's influence in his life. This is because these mantras are closely related with powerful divine energies. If the deities associated with these energies are invited, they require the practitioner's system to be properly aligned, so that it may properly host these energies. If the prerequisites are not met, chanting these mantras can cause serious adverse effects, including psychological disturbances for both the practitioner and those around him. This is poorly understood today and is, in part, due to misunderstanding the power of Saṃskṛta as it relates to yoga.

Given that pronunciation is the key to the life of mantra, it should not be underestimated. I can recall an incident when I was a Saṃskṛta student at the *pāṭhaśālā,* or traditional school, at Shringeri, Karnataka, near my birthplace in southern India. There were nine of us students sitting around our noble teacher, Śrī Ganesha Shastry. Śrī Ganesha Shastry was a spiritually disciplined man known for his knowledge of Saṃskṛta and Āyurveda. By nature, he was very kind, affectionate, and loving toward us students. He would recite a few words or sentences in Saṃskṛta, and we were expected to repeat the same lines the next day. However, if even a single word was mispronounced, Śrī Ganesha Shastry would get angry. He would exclaim, "Oh, you have mispronounced this word. You have not only created a wrong impression in your mind, but you have caused wrong impressions to me as well as these eight classmates! Now, how can this be eliminated?"

As a punishment, the student would have to pronounce the word correctly ten times. The purpose of this was to establish a correct, right impression and, to some extent, decrease the previous wrong impression. In those days, those who often mispronounced words might even receive slaps on the thighs with a bamboo stick!

THE POWER OF DEVOTION

Laukika mantra requires less precision. It derives its impact from the amount of devotion that we bring to our chanting. The sound of the mantra is simply a means to carry our devotion to the deity. Therefore, a laukika mantra can be given to anybody, because devotion is the key.

Providing a practitioner brings a sufficient level of devotion, lack of proper pronunciation will not hinder its effectiveness or cause adverse impacts.

In India it is typically regarded as disrespectful for one person's feet to touch another person. However, if a small baby comes to us with a full expression of love, we do not mind where his hands or feet touch. A baby can even stand on top of us and we will not feel disrespected. In the same way, if the practitioner's love and devotion are sincere while chanting laukika mantras, the deity will overlook any mispronunciation. In laukika mantra, devotion is enough.

APPENDIX TWO

Sanskrit Pronunciation Guide

VOWELS

a	"a" as in "father"
ā	"aah" as in "aah"
i	"ee" as in "meek"
ī	"eee" as in "eeek"
u	"oo" as in "brood"
ū	"ooo" as in "boo"
ṛ	"ru" as in "rude"
e	"ay" as in "day"
ai	"ie" as in ""die"
o	"oe" as in "doe"
au	"ow" as in "cow"

CONSONANTS

k, g, t, d, j, p, b	These are all pronounced as they appear.
c	"ch" as in "charge"
ṭ, ḍ, ṇ, ṣ	These are retroflex consonants, where the tongue curls back and touches the roof of the mouth. There is no English equivalent. For example, "ṭ" is like "t," except the tongue touches the roof of the mouth, rather than behind the teeth.
kh, gh, ch, jh, ṭh, ḍh, th, dh, ph, bh	These are aspirated consonants. They are pronounced with a push of breath, or aspiration.

NASALS

ṅ	"ng" as in "ring"
ñ	"ny" as in "canyon"
ṇ	"ṇ" as in "guṇa" Retroflex (see above); no English equivalent.
n	"n" as in "no"
m	"m" as in "mow"

SILIBANTS

s	"s" as in "save"
ś	"sh" as in "shave"
ṣ	as in "doṣa." This has no English equivalent; it is similar to "sh," except that it is retroflex.

SEMI-VOWELS

y, r, l, v	These are pronounced similarly to the English equivalent.

ANUSVĀRA

ṃ	The anusvāra is a nasalization that approximates "m," as in "Saṃskṛta"

VISARGA

ḥ	The visarga is an added aspiration, often at the end of the word, that incorporates the preceding vowel. Thus, "namaḥ" is pronounced, "namaha," "hariḥ" is pronounced, "harihi."

Index

attachment (*continued*)
diminishing obstacle of, 242–43
duty and, 64–65
to Eternal Truth, 135–36
love and, 65–66
to possessions, 134, 135
See also aparigraha (detachment from possessions)
austerity. *See* tapas (austerity)
avadhūta, 266
Āyurveda, 12, 47, 93, 153, 157, 164, 168, 169, 218, 228

bathing
before meals, 178–79
before practice, 196, 197
Bhagavad-Gītā, 82, 166, 231–32
Bhakti Yoga, 68, 69, 73, 74, 291–94
bhoga, 19, 21, 23, 116
birth and conception
aśauca and, 199, 201
brahmacarya and, 126–28
Eternal Truth and, 24
in support of liberation, 124–25
blessings
of Nature, 244–45, 247–48
truthful speaking and, 97
bliss
contentment and, 212–13
mahat state and, 32, 33
as powerful antidote, 22
of Samādhi, 17–27, 48, 49, 71, 212, 266
as ultimate goal, xi, 11, 12
vs. worldly happiness, 18–19
See also happiness
body
āsana and, 79
cleanliness and, 203–4
as gateway within, 43
as unimaginable vehicle, 40, 49–50
See also mind and body; physical constitution
Brahma, 117, 120, 169
brahmacāris, 118, 119, 124, 161
brahmacarya (moving toward Eternal Truth), 63, 116–30
conception and, 126–28
explanation of, 117–18
marriage and family and, 124–25, 126–28
Nature's principles and, 125–26, 127, 128
sexuality and, 118–19, 123–24, 125, 128–30
stages of life and, 119–20
youth and, 120–23
Brahmasūtra, 231
breath
prāṇāyāma and, 79, 289
problems with air and, 189
union of prāṇa and apāna, 36
buddhi, 32, 38

cāndrāyaṇa, 218
celibacy, 117, 119
chanting
before meals, 176
as tapas, 218, 222–23
See also japa (chanting)
citta, 32
cleanliness. *See* śauca (physical cleanliness)
compassion
cultivating, 94
dayā and, 138–40
sattvic energy and, 43
contentment. *See* santoṣa (contentment)
cursing, 85, 86, 97

three main paths in, 68–73, 285–94
as union of prakṛti into puruṣa, 36
as union of prāṇa and apāna, 36
Yoga Sūtras, 23, 29, 30, 82, 83, 130, 138, 225, 228
Yogi Yājñavalkya, 82, 83
yogic education, 264–65
yogic experiences
absence of, 14–15, 24
effects on health, 46–48
memory and, 45–46
naturalness of, 13, 15
recognizing, 24–26
surrendering worldly pleasure and, 23
yogic sight, 20, 45–46, 236, 237
youth
food for, 160–61
sexuality and, 120–23

About the Author

Dr. Shankaranarayana Jois began his study of Saṃskṛta at the early age of five. Later, he attended the Maharaja's Government Saṃskṛta College at Mysore, India, where he acquired a qualification as Vidwan in Literary Criticism and Indian Logic. He also completed his MA in Saṃskṛta and a PhD in yoga. Dr. Jois holds a degree in Hindi and is qualified as Pandit in Kannada, the state language of Karnataka. He retired from the Saṃskṛta College of Mysore as assistant professor in 2002. He is the founder and a trustee of Bharati Yoga Dhama, an organization dedicated to the preservation of ancient Indian arts and sciences, including the divine language, Saṃskṛta. Dr. Jois is also deeply knowledgeable in Vedic astrology through a hereditary link. Most influential in Dr. Jois's life has been the teachings of his Eternal Teacher, Śrī Raṅga Mahāguru (1913–1969), a highly honored Enlightened yogi who had deep insight into the Truth behind the original Indian sciences. For feedback, comments, or questions please visit http://sadvidyafoundation.org.